RUNNING A PRACTICE

Running a Practice

A MANUAL OF PRACTICE MANAGEMENT

THIRD EDITION

R.V.H. JONES, K.J. BOLDEN,
D.J. PEREIRA GRAY and M.S. Hall

CROOM HELM
London • New York • Sydney

Reprinted 1981, 1983 and 1984

Reprinted 1987

Croom Helm Ltd, Provident House, Burrell Row,
Beckenham, Kent, BR3 1AT
Croom Helm Australia, 44-50 Waterloo Road,
North Ryde, 2113, New South Wales

British Library Cataloguing in Publication Data

Running a practice: a manual of practice management. — 3rd ed.
1. Medical offices — Great Britain — Management 2. Family medicine — Great Britain
I. Jones, R.V.H.
362.1'72'068 R728

ISBN 0-7099-1455-5 Pbk

Published in the USA by
Croom Helm
in association with Methuen, Inc.
29 West 35th Street
New York, NY 10001

Library of Congress Cataloging-in-Publication Data

Running a practice.

Includes bibliographies and index.
1. Family medicine — Practice — Great Britain.
2. Physicians (general practice) — Great Britain.
3. Medical Offices — Great Britain — Management.
I. Jones, R.V.H. (Robert Vernon Holmes)
R729.5.G4R86 1985 610'.68 84-23840

ISBN 0-7099-1455-5 Pbk

Typeset by Leaper & Gard Ltd, Bristol
Printed and bound in Great Britain by
Biddles Ltd, Guildford and King's Lynn

CONTENTS

ACKNOWLEDGEMENTS

We should like to express our gratitude to the following for their help and advice: Professor G. Duncan Mitchell, Professor of Sociology, University of Exeter; Dr Trevor Hoskins, Hon. Sec. of the Medical Officers of Schools Association; Dr D Buchanan, Scottish Secretary of the British Medical Association; N.O.J. Holberton, Devon Family Practitioner Committee and D. Mullins, chartered accountant.

We should also like to record our appreciation of the advice and helpful criticism given by Drs J.A.S. Forman, S. Jane Richards and Peter Selley.

We are grateful to the editors of *Update* and of the *Journal of the Royal College of General Practitioners* for permission to publish those parts of the chapter on the independent contractor which have already appeared in these journals.

Finally our secretaries, especially Mrs Avis Hilder, who have survived indecipherable tapes and indescribable writing, deserve our grateful thanks.

PREFACE

As part of the Vocational Training Scheme at Exeter trainees are offered a practice management course during their final year. Originally planned as a practical course it was soon found necessary to explain the philosophy which underlies the working arrangements and decision-making in our own practices. The lack of reference material for such a course has prompted the production of this book. As we take joint responsibility for the views expressed, chapters have not been attributed to individuals.

We hope that trainees, trainers, and possibly others, may find something of interest.

Preface to the Second Edition

The preparation of a second edition has enabled us to correct some errors, to revise and expand the chapters on records and audit, and to introduce new chapters on practice accounts and the training practice.

We hope that the usefulness of the book as an introduction to practice management will have been enhanced.

Preface to the Third Edition

General practice is continually changing, adapting and developing. Over the past few years awareness of the need to understand the roles and skills of health visitors, social workers, nurses and therapists has increased. Emphasis has been placed on prevention, and more preventive procedures have been undertaken in practices. More attention has been paid to recalling patients for regular surveillance. More computers have been installed. The fact that when practices increase in size and complexity changes in management method are essential if confusion and inefficiency are to be avoided has become more widely appreciated.

At the same time there has been a shift from theory to action. In our visits to practices round the country we have become aware that management changes are not just being discussed, they are happening. The preparation of a third edition has given us the opportunity to reflect these developments.

Finally, as the number of appendices multiplied it seemed more convenient to attach them to the appropriate chapters as a second section. We hope they will be useful to secretaries and receptionists as well as to practitioners.

R.V.H.J.
K.J.B.
D.J.P.G.
M.S.H.

INTRODUCTION

The title phrase 'running a practice' was chosen to indicate that the contents of this book would be an overall view of all those activities which are involved in the day-to-day and longer-term organisation of a practice within the National Health Service. This is a large and complex subject. We have deliberately chosen to concentrate on principles rather than detail so that consideration can be given to all major topics within a relatively small volume. Some examples and summaries will be found in the supplementary section to each chapter where appropriate. Detailed descriptions of office procedures have been given by Drury and in a booklet distributed by the General Medical Services Committee.

For a general practitioner the ability to run his practice efficiently has certain direct and obvious advantages. He knows where he is — the surgeries are not overbooked, all forms and equipment are to hand, he can plan his half-days and holidays, the accounts are straightforward and up to date. His income is higher, with claim forms for items of service being filled in correctly and submitted without delay, mileage allowances are noted, bills are paid and reimbursements claimed at times which increase cash flow. The atmosphere in which he works is pleasant and friendly.

There are, however, other advantages for patients and doctors which are not so immediately apparent. Practice management and organisation are usually considered as distinct from clinical care. When lectures are given or courses are held for general practitioners the subject matter is either clinical or practice management. Rarely is any connection made between the two. Yet there is a direct relationship. Poor management inevitably results in a lower standard of clinical care. If staff are unhappy with their contracts (or lack of them), if partners are unhappy about their working conditions and do not meet to agree how things might be improved, if requests for visits are mislaid, messages lost, forms not available or wrongly filled in, the frustration and unhappiness in the practice spills over into relationships with patients. If through lack of organisation doctors are rushed or their surgeries are impossibly full, they become resentful and the care their patients receive is bound to suffer. If records are a shambles patients may be in danger of being given a drug to which they are sensitive, or a child fail to receive a booster because his immunisation state is unrecorded.

There is no doubt in our minds that in order to deliver a high standard of clinical care, clinical work must be backed up by good practice organisation.

There is also no doubt that one of the skills of practice management is to make sure that in spite of its complexity the practice runs smoothly, that the hum of activity arising from the organisation should be inaudible to the patient. If, as we believe, general practice should provide each patient with continuing personal care, it should be in a friendly, calm atmosphere in which as far as possible the patient feels at ease and at home. Hustle, bustle and over-busyness diminish patients. One aim of a patient-orientated practice should be to keep its necessarily complex organisation out of sight. In the following pages we describe the various behind-the-scenes activities which are involved in running a practice within the National Health Service.

References

Drury, M. *The Medical Secretary's Handbook*, 4th Edition (London: Ballière Tindall, 1981)

The Business of General Practice 1983/84, 3rd Edition. Prepared by General Practitioner and Medeconomics for the General Medical Services Committee.

PART ONE:

THE SCENE

1 THE NATURE OF GENERAL PRACTICE

There are two main kinds of doctor: those who are primarily interested in diseases and those who are primarily interested in people. Perhaps the most important decision of all for any young doctor, before, during and after qualification, is to identify his own characteristics and to become quite certain in which category he or she is. Both types of doctor are essential for the future of medical practice. Both undertake equally valuable work.

For the disease-centred doctor the kind of disease the patient has is the central focus of his interest and care, and the particular person who happens to have it is inevitably the secondary consideration. By contrast for patient-centred doctors the patient, his personality, his attitudes, his family and home are of central interest and the particular kind of disease he happens to have at the time is important but secondary.

The crucial importance of this distinction is that doctors in one category usually do not feel completely at home if they are practising the other branch of medicine.

Most trainees if they are undertaking a three-year programme of training for general practice will have already decided that they are patient-centred doctors. Many will have doubts, however, and some will have serious misgivings. It is important that these are voiced and discussed.

Variety in General Practice

People sometimes talk about general practice as if it is a uniform whole, which can be discussed and debated as if it has fixed and common characteristics. The opposite is of course the case and one of the main characteristics of general practice is its extreme diversity. No two practices are quite the same and even in the same road adjacent practices may have totally different attitudes and standards.

All those entering general practice must begin to understand some of the reasons for the variety. These conveniently come under the headings of: people, place, premises, partner(s) and personality.

1. People

Medicine is a service. The purpose of medical care is to bring to the people in any society a medical service appropriate to their needs. It follows that the first essential in considering any health system is to test the appropriateness of the service in relation to the needs of the people as perceived by themselves and by the health professionals. This principle holds true in general practice and one of the main causes of variety in general practice is the variety of people themselves. Obvious examples are race, social class, and age structure.

Race. Culture has an immense influence on attitudes towards illness and on attitudes to the process of seeking help. The presence of significant numbers of people of a different race as patients will have a major impact on the pattern of a general practice. Changes in the racial pattern of the locality will alter the character of the practices in that locality.

Social Class. The tremendous significance of social class in relation to illness is little appreciated from hospitals, but there is overwhelming evidence that social class is one of the main determinants of morbidity, mortality, and the use of health services. Life expectation at every age is significantly less in the lower social classes from the perinatal period to old age. People in social class five on average die younger than those in social class one. In analysing the people who are the patients in a practice, the numbers and properties and the different social classes greatly influence the nature of the work in that practice (DHSS, 1976).

Age. Similarly, the age of a patient is another major determinant of illness (Fry, 1977). Not only do elderly people often develop several disabilities simultaneously but their increasing loss of independence, frailty and loss of mobility mean that they have a disproportionately high home visiting rate. In some practices on the south coast of England the proportion of all patients who are over the age of 65 is more than one third whereas in other towns it may be as low as 5 per cent. The distribution of age of the patients of the practice therefore is another cause of variety in general practice.

2. The Place

General practice has long been close to the people and indeed is a community service in a community setting. All general practices to some extent absorb the pattern of living of people in that area and hence there are wide variations between practices in, say, a Welsh mining village, the centre of Liverpool, and a practice on Dartmoor. Because the problems of people's lives impinge on us and indeed may dominate, the problems of people living in different places will be reflected in the general practitioner's consulting room. The place where the practice *is* will inevitably determine to a large extent the pattern of practice.

3. Provision

Although general practice may be the most isolated and individual medical branch of the health service, general practitioners do not practise alone. The quality of the work that they can do, whether in single-handed practice or a big partnership, must always depend to a considerable extent on the provision of other health services in the neighbourhood. Whether or not there is a general-practitioner hospital, whether or not there is a general-practitioner maternity unit, whether or not the local social services department is coping well with its workload, whether or not the provision of health visitors and nurses is adequate, will govern the use by practitioners of these services and hence their pattern of practice. In understanding how, and why, a practice works and what its potential is for further improvement, the provision of other health and social services in the neighbourhood must therefore be taken into consideration.

4. Premises

The premises used for general medical practice changed little in the nineteenth century, but a dramatic revolution occurred in the middle of the twentieth century. One of the most obvious signs of this radical review of primary care was the transformation of general-practitioner premises. It can now be seen that getting the premises correct was rightly one of the first targets for the reorganisation of general practice that took place in the 1960s (BMA Charter, 1965).

Whatever the skills, hopes, attitudes, or aspirations of the doctor he needs a place to exercise his skills. For example, if there is no treatment room it is difficult to realise the full potential of both attached nurses and practice nurses. The simple criterion of whether or not there is a treatment room is one of the great indicators of the range of activities which can take place in practices. Many practices without treatment rooms will refer to hospital conditions which doctors and nurses working together can often manage, and manage excellently, in a properly equipped nursing sister's room.

The presence of a common room can similarly subtly alter the relationships between partners and other members of general-practice teams. The Scottish Council for Postgraduate Medical Education (1977) lists the presence of a common room as one of the factors now expected in training practices. They believe that the presence of a library in the common room and the ability of partners to meet on neutral ground is of special value in promoting partnership discussion and relationships. It is not, of course, true that without a common room partners cannot meet and discuss; in many such practices close partnership relationships exist. Nevertheless, in our experience having a room where partners can meet independently of another partner being held up and running late, or having to fit in an extra patient or medical, is a great boon; it promotes relaxed discussion over coffee and may be a convenient setting for regular meetings of partners and, say, a weekly lunch. Such meetings are particularly important in bigger partnerships.

It is difficult to assess how irritating it can be if partners do not have their own consulting rooms, which is still the case in many general practices today. Practices which have been able to provide each partner with a separate room make it possible for consulting rooms to be furnished much more personally, and for them to reflect the personality of the doctor.

Finally, there is no doubt that many of the future developments in general practice will depend upon improved methods of record-keeping and the introduction of new systems of organisation of records including, for example, such basic methods as age/sex registers and diagnostic indexes. All these systems take up room and it is becoming clear that those practices which have enough room to organise efficient systems of handling information are becoming able to offer a better standard of care for their patients. It follows that the presence of an adequate size secretarial office, or better still a second office, may be a condition for improving the standard of clinical care.

5. Partners

We analyse in Chapter 12 the significance of the partnership relationship to general practitioners. Of all the factors involved in choosing a new practice, we advise trainees to place the greatest weight on being sure of compatibility of personality with partners. The partnership relationship is a form of professional marriage, and there is no doubt that the ability to practise a high standard of clinical care depends on the quality of care, the attitude and the standard of one's partners. Even in those practices in which separate lists are maintained, and in which patients identify with a particular partner, it is always true that there will be some crossover between partners and patients and inevitably partners will see one's patients in the evenings, during holidays and study leave. Furthermore, partners will be responsible for forming the philosophy of the practice which will influence and outwardly govern the attitudes and behaviour of the practice secretaries, receptionists, and the health visitor and nurses. The feeling of the group of partners which is so difficult to express is the average picture that the partners convey to their working colleagues.

No matter what the ideals and skills of a new incoming partner, the ultimate effect he will have on his patients will be determined to an extent greater than he perhaps realises by the other partners in the practice. Furthermore, in a close working relationship over the years, partners increasingly influence each other. There is no reasonable hope of expecting to change two or three senior partners in their views. They are much more likely to change the views of the lonely isolated incoming partner. The tradition and history of a practice has a strong influence on its organisation and philosophy. The presence of different practice traditions is a further factor underlying the variety found in general practice.

6. The Doctor's Personality

One of the landmarks of modern general practice was the publication of Balint's book, *The Doctor, His Patient and the Illness* in 1957. It has been said (*Journal of the Royal College of General Practitioners*, 1972) 'Balint will become for general practice what Freud has become for psychiatry', that is to say he will be seen as a great prophet who introduced a major new dimension to a discipline.

Whilst it is absurd to suggest the psychoanalytical approach of Freud is the 'be all and end all' of psychiatry, it is impossible to deny that the whole development of modern psychiatry has been influenced by his views.

Similarly, it is quite possible to agree that much of modern general practice does not depend upon Balint, but it is equally impossible to deny that his views have influenced, and decisively influenced, the last twenty-five years of development of the discipline of general practice.

One of the key ideas which Balint introduced was that much of the care provided in general practice depended on the personality of the doctor himself. He expressed this in the model by saying that the doctor was the most important 'drug' used in general practice; and followed it through by saying that doctors who wished to practise family medicine must learn to understand their own personalities, to understand the side-effects of the use of this drug, and the indications for appropriate use. Even nearly thirty years later this message has not yet been generally understood. Many general practitioners still enter general practice, having attended courses of vocational training without learning this essential fact. In order to be good general practitioners we must first understand ourselves. We must understand the strength and weakness of our own personalities, the way we affect other people, and the way we cope with some of our more important inner feelings.

There are many ways of obtaining these insights, but the simplest and most effective appears to be by a series of discussions with one's peers, preferably led by someone who is experienced in the analysis of personality and inter-personal behaviour. The traditional psychoanalytical school believed that general practitioners obtained these insights best if led by a professionally trained psychoanalyst, such as Balint himself, and this school has continued until the present time. Others have increasingly wondered if general practitioners could not themselves lead groups and assist their colleagues in obtaining similar insights.

Many vocational training schemes are now firmly based on the concept of continuing small group discussion as an essential method of helping trainees understand their own personality. By working with a group of colleagues, by arguing and struggling with knowledge, ideas and attitudes, trainees over a long period of time (preferably three years) begin to understand the importance of human behaviour, learn to tolerate their colleagues' idiosyncrasies, and more important still begin to understand how their colleagues tolerate them.

These insights we believe are essential if a general practitioner is to be able to cope with the tremendous variety of behaviour which will be presented to him by patients who are, or think they may be, ill. Without such training, anger in the doctor is common, and it is striking how angry trainees or young principals may become when patients behave in ways they have hitherto assumed were inappropriate. Only by facing such behaviour among one's peers can one learn to recognise patterns which make the doctor angry, and begin to understand a patient's feelings. Among the educational aims of the Exeter course learning to feel what it is like to be a patient is one of the highest on the list.

Recordon (1972) has said that doctors eventually get the patients that they deserve, and it is probably true that over a period of at least a dozen years or more there will be a progressive trend for patients of certain types and categories to collect on any particular doctor's list. In order to understand this phenomenon it is necessary to understand the personality of the general practitioner. If, for example, he has a particular interest in a particular disease, whether organic or psychological, he is likely to detect it earlier and to treat it more effectively if only because he is more interested and gives more of himself. He tends to collect patients with such a condition by recommendation and referral. If, on the other hand, he is uncomfortable with patients who express anger or fear, he will over the years gradually lose such patients, or lose contact with them as they seek the outlets they need from other doctors or other sources. Thus over a period of time the doctor will see more and more of what he is interested in, and less and less of what he is least efficient at detecting or managing.

Whilst this may lead to contentment over the years, it can also lead to a fall in standards if the doctor is not confronted periodically with evidence of those aspects of care in which he still has most to learn. Developing a tolerant partnership relationship is one of the ways in which the small group of the partners meeting together may be able to assist each other in such aspects of medicine.

Most doctors have inner needs to dominate people, and may succeed in establishing dominant relationships with large numbers of their patients. Others have a need to be loved, and will over the years collect large numbers of patients who will fulfil this emotional need. Ultimately each general practitioner must ask himself the question whether or not he needs to be respected, or needs to be loved; most of us fall into one or other of these categories. This can be a helpful analysis in aiding a young doctor to determine in which aspects of care he or she is likely to be relatively strong or weak.

The personality of the doctor is thus of special importance. It is the key to successful personal medical care. The variety found among general practitioner's personalities is one of the main causes of the variety found in general practice.

References and Further Reading

Balint, M. *The Doctor, His Patient and the Illness*, 2nd edition (London: Pitman, 1964).

British Medical Association Charter (London: BMA, 1965).

Department of Health and Social Security. *Prevention and Health: Everybody's Business* (London: HMSO, 1976).

Fry, J. James Mackenzie Lecture 1976. *Journal of the Royal College of General Practitioners*, 26 (1977), pp. 9-17.

Journal of the Royal College of General Practitioners. Editorial, Michael Balint. 22 (1972), pp. 133-5.

Recordon, P. *Journal of the Royal College of General Practitioners*, 22 (1972). pp. 818-27.

Scottish Council for Postgraduate Medical Education. *Training in General Practice* (Edinburgh: SCPME, 1977).

2 THE GENERAL PRACTITIONER AS AN INDEPENDENT CONTRACTOR

Many of the characteristics found in general practice in this country today are based on the fact that general practitioners are independent contractors. A simple definition is that an independent contractor is a self employed person who agrees (contracts) to provide a service for someone else either himself or through his employees. Self employed lawyers, dentists, plumbers, opticians, typists are all independent contractors.

Being an independent contractor a general practitioner has the freedom to organise his own business as he deems appropriate. But with this freedom goes administrative and financial responsibility for the business and responsibility for the service he provides. If general practitioners were salaried employees this book would not have been written.

Because there is still confusion over the implications of independent contractor status for general practice, because present-day practice is based upon it, and because it has been and still is a controversial issue within the National Health Service, we have devoted this chapter to comparing the salaried system with the independent contractor system and discussing the related advantages and disadvantages

Salaried System

The salaried system leads inevitably to hierarchies because it is rare in human groups or organisations for one person to be able to relate to or control more than about 15 others. Once an organisation grows beyond this number the tendency is for a series of ranks to emerge, each with defined responsibility for the rank below. In its most fully developed form the salaried system tends towards a 'bureaucracy' (a system of offices arranged in rank order); examples include the Civil Service, the police and the hospital medical and nursing services.

Advantages

There are many advantages in a salaried system. By employing a person the employer has control and can direct the work. The employee has a defined contract, usually defined conditions of service, and these are often comparable with those of others in similar grades. Additional advantages to the staff include interchangeability of benefits and terms of service. There are usually other privileges such as sick pay, defined periods of notice, pensions, and moving allowances.

Some eighteenth-century social scientists regarded the bureaucracy as the most logical system of organising men. In the perfect system promotion would be by merit and each man would rise to exactly the point in the hierarchy most suitable for his talents. The whole would thus co-ordinate the abilities of all the individuals in the organisation to the best possible effect. Such ideas remain common today. There are still many people who favour the tidy, logical, structured approach to organisation found in salaried systems.

Another important advantage of salaried systems is consistency. A team organised in this way can be relied upon to provide services consistently. It is no accident that most big organisations, whether governmental like the Civil Service or private like the banks or universities, adopt a bureaucratic structure.

Salaried servants are freed from the burden of financial involvement with the enterprise. It is for the employer to provide the premises, equipment and payments — only rarely is there any question of the employee participating in the capital. This usually relieves employees from having to borrow in order to buy a share in the firm.

Disadvantages

The price of this system lies in three main characteristics: impersonality, lack of consumer choice, and diminution of the individual within the system. Impersonality is inevitable: indeed, big systems are built on the assumption that the system or firm is more important than the individual. Big organisations must discourage individuality except among those of the highest ranks. People who break the rules cause extra work — eccentricities are expensive.

Lack of consumer choice tends to follow from the standardisation and the authority of the arrangements. It is hard to choose one's police sergeant, ward sister, hospital house officer or local government officer — the individual client is expected to fit in with the system.

Diminution of the individual follows from the rules and regulations of the system. Salaried employment means by definition that, in the words of the Courts, a 'master/servant relationship' is deemed to exist. There can be no escape from this authority, which enables the employer or the superior in the hierarchy to give orders – the recipient has to accept or leave. Apart from the direct authority, there is usually a considerable amount of indirect authority: decision-taking is controlled. Each person is usually allocated a range of decisions (up to a defined figure or degree of importance) after which responsibility has to be referred upwards. This system ensures quality control through a good degree of regulation and supervision and acts to protect the client against error or incompetence. While it is perfectly possible for individuals to feel fulfilled within hierarchies, there is a tendency for these constraints to inhibit the person and to discourage originality, flamboyance, or an irregular solution to problems. Standardisation, while protecting quality, may limit initiative.

Independent Contractor System

Individuals or groups of individuals who agree to do something for someone else in return for payment or in exchange for some other service are independent contractors. Essentially, the system is the agreement to provide a service. In law, the independent contractor has a contract *for* services, compared with a salaried employee who has a contract *of* service. The independent contractor retains his independence. Furthermore, the word 'agreement' emphasises that there is always some element of negotiation between the contractor and the person who is the customer or who commands the service.

Independent contractors are commonplace in society, and their numbers may now be growing. They include all shopkeepers, businessmen, advisers, private consultants, and those who offer services such as typing.

Most, but not all, professional people are independent contractors, including dentists, pharmacists, solicitors, barristers, accountants, surveyors and general practitioners in all Western societies. Jones (1978) showed that general practice across Western Europe worked within an independent contract. Ever since 1911/12 British general practitioners have consistently chosen an independent contract and have opposed a salaried service. This is still the policy of the Conference of Local Medical Committees. General practitioners thus like to see themselves as part of a local community and comparable in it to other independent professional people.

The features and characteristics of independent contractors are (a) flexibility, (b) variability in provision, (c) emphasis on the personality of the contractor, and (d) emphasis on the supplier/client relationship.

Advantages

Flexibility refers to the way in which arrangements are provided. Shops may open late, offer home deliveries, or decide whether or not to offer credit, all of which may be dramatically different from an institution of the same kind next door. Personal incentives are quite common. They can take the form of fees or commission and may be considerable — a barrister can earn more than the prime minister.

The independent contract depends upon and seeks to exploit the personality of the contractor. Independent contractors like to be involved with customers. They value personal relationships with clients and a long-term view. They are sensitive to the collective opinion of their clients or patients.

Independent contractors value people as people. It is usual for the contractor to use his or her own name, to have it on the front door and usually on the firm's writing paper. Personal eccentricities are not only tolerated — they are often exploited.

Disadvantages

Standards vary and are less well controlled. Quality of goods or services may differ markedly and will tend to depend on the personality of the people involved. Standard setting is often a problem for independent contractors, in both the business and professional world, and arrangements appear untidy.

A further problem arising from the variability of arrangements may be low pay and poor conditions for employees. This is the other side of the coin of incentives. Some independent contractors and their employees work long hours for poor rewards.

Sociological Analysis

Sociologists have analysed these features of salaried and independent contractor systems and have concluded that they can act as determinants of behaviour. Structure (sociological) can thus determine process (behaviour).

The term 'spiralist' is used to describe a person travelling up a hierarchy. Such people are usually bureaucrats as defined above. They achieve promotion by passing examinations and often move periodically for promotion. They are very conscious of and dependent upon supervisers for references. Sometimes they may value the system rather than the client.

'Burgess', by contrast, is a term used to describe those who settle in a locality. They tend to identify with the community with whom they live and serve and are not expert or seek promotion. They make their money by local personal relationships; they allow standards of goods or service to slip at times.

Influence on Medical Behaviour

Susser and Watson (1971), in a standard textbook of sociology, carry this analysis further. In a well-known passage they contrast the advantages and disadvantages of these two systems. In some ways the strengths and weaknesses of the two systems are reciprocal to each other.

> Typically, the staff consider the patient in hospital with necessary if concerned detachment, as a case and an object of scientific study. Decisions about management of the case must display technical competence and be justifiable to colleagues on scientific grounds. The hospital 'encapsulates' the patient, whose set of associations and ideas are thereby strictly limited, and the behaviour expected from him is accepting, submissive, and dependent. His needs tend to be assessed within this restricted framework. Thus decisions about him are often made with perfunctory attention to the latest roles he has relinquished in the world outside, in family, work, and leisure, and he cannot appeal to those outside for support.

On the other hand, Susser and Watson continue:

> The pressures in the community situation of the practitioner

> direct his attention to the personal needs of his patients, but they may isolate him professionally and preclude constant reference to the scientific judgement of colleagues.

They conclude:

> The pressures in the hospital situation of the specialist maintain his technical competence and divert his attention from the personal needs of patients ... The mistakes of general practice often seem to arise from technical failures; the mistakes of hospital practice often do so from failures of communication.

These analyses by professional sociologists are helpful in clarifying the conflicts which surround these systems. One of the difficulties is that those politically to the left of centre tend to favour salaried systems — which logically appeal to those who support equality as a moral issue and who like ordered arrangements. On the other hand, those to the right of centre tend to favour independent contracts, as these emphasise and encourage initiative, provide incentives, and cater more for the individual.

British General Practice

British general practice provides a fascinating case study, but is a complex and in many ways an atypical example.

General practitioners are independent contractors and are self-employed for the purposes of income tax. It can be seen that most of the broad features described above fit fairly well. General practitioners are burgesses, they look to their local community and do not seek promotion by moving, as do spiralists. They are very dependent on relationships and recommendations. Services are flexible and arrangements in remote rural practices are almost unrecognisable compared with some inner city practices. Practitioners have great discretion and choice in the way they provide services, and patients can choose and change their doctor (about 1% of the population do so each year).

On the other hand, ever since 1948 the General Medical Services Committee has negotiated a series of changes to the general practitioner's contract that have had the cumulative effect of bringing the total package nearer to a salaried system. Sick pay, inflation-protected pensions and monthly advances are all examples. Health centres exclude problems of financial involvement in the premises and are welcomed by about one-fifth of practitioners. However, four-fifths of British practitioners prefer, for one reason or another, to own their own premises.

In terms of financial involvement, it can be argued that British general practitioners have a negative incentive to invest in equipment in that they have to pay the whole cost but are not entitled to a return on use. However, one favourable feature is the keen awareness of costs that practitioners have to acquire. At a time when it is being suggested that hospital clinicians should become 'budget-holders' to help them acquire such understanding, it is notable that general practitioner principals, by virtue of this system, are budget-holders automatically.

One of the advantages of a salaried system is consistency of service. It is interesting to note the efforts which are being made within the profession itself to raise standards and provide a consistent service while remaining within the independent contractor system.

Summing Up

That the independent contractor status of the general practitioners is still a controversial issue is undoubted (Tudor Hart and Pereira Gray, 1984). We believe that the crucial difference between the philosophy of the supporters of the two systems lies in the importance they place on personal relationships.

Those who follow Balint (1964), and the belief that the human aspects of the doctor/patient relationship are central, will believe that the balance must tilt towards some version of an independent contract. Impersonality must threaten personal care.

Moreover, general practice is built on relationships, both legal and practical. Co-operation, with mutual respect and support from partners, is a good basis on which to build relationships with patients, which should also be based on co-operation, mutual respect, and support. Modern general practice emphasises the role of the patient as a respected equal partner in consultation, and by implication emphasises negotiation as a way of professional life. It is logical, therefore, for general practitioners themselves to work within a negotiated contract for services, rather than in hierarchies.

If in the future general practice were to move away from a personal caring service towards a highly technical service, then the case for a salaried service would become more logical.

References and Further Reading

Balint, M. *The Doctor, His Patient and the Illness*, 2nd ed. (London: Pitman, 1964).

Jones, R.V.H. *General Practice in the E.E.C. Update*, 16 (1978) pp. 1503-15.

Susser, M.W., Watson, W. *Sociology in Medicine*, 2nd ed. (London: OUP, 1971), p. 189.

Tudor Hart, J. and Pereira Gray, D.J. Letters: 'Independent Contractors and Salaried Servants', *Update*, 29 (1984), p. 167.

Chapter 2: Section 2

Tabular presentation of comparison between the characteristics of independent contractors and salaried employees in bureaucracies

Characteristic	Independent Contractor	Salaried Employee
1. General characteristic	Variety Self-employed Administratively untidy Variable standard of service	Uniformity Employee Administratively tidy 'Master/servant' order
2. Sociological classification	Burgess	Some are spiralists
3. Authority	General — often employs staff Can never be given orders Negotiators	Specific — accountable upwards and authority over subordinates 'Officers/supervisors'
4. Philosophy	Flexible and great freedom to negotiate local arrangements	Rules, often nationally determined Consistency and standardisation of policy
5. Personality of operator	Individuality encouraged Use of names and relationships with clients valued	Individuality discouraged Anonymity of staff Correspondence to junior members of hierarchy discouraged

6. Contract	Contract for services	Contract of service
7. Pay	Usually not incremental salary scale Often some element of fee for service or commission	Salary by definition Usually incremental scale
8. Premises and equipment	Usually responsible for providing own premises	Usually provided by the employing authority
9. Staffing	Usually responsible for own holidays, locum, and pension	Employer responsible for holiday arrangements, locums, and often pension
10. Retirement	Variable Individual negotiation	Usually compulsory at fixed age
11. Partnership(s)	Common 'Jointly and severally' responsible in law and for tax and partners' debts	Rare No responsibility for colleagues' taxes or debts
12. Income tax assessed under	Schedule D 'wholly and exclusively'	Schedule E, PAYE 'wholly and necessarily'
13. Responsibility	Ultimately answerable to client/patient	Ultimately answerable to superior or employer
14. Professional negligence	Professional is solely responsible and alone can be sued	Employing authority responsible and can be sued (as well as or instead of professional)
15. Degree of choice by client/patient	Usually wide choice and relatively easy to change	Little or no choice of individual or department Difficult to change

Source: Gray, D.J. Pereira. 'General Practitioners and the Independent Contractor Status', *Journal of the Royal College of General Practitioners*, 27 (1977), pp. 750-6.

PART TWO:

PEOPLE

3 INDIVIDUALS AND ROLES

History

The concept of the general-practice team developed only slowly. Certainly until the middle of the twentieth century the most common form of practice was that of a single doctor working, often with his wife to help him as secretary, with minimal or even no supporting staff at all. The doctor usually worked from his own house. District nurses and midwives worked in a district (employed initially by voluntary bodies, more recently by the Local Authority) and were not connected formally with practices in any way.

The first supporting staff to be recruited were receptionists followed in quick succession by secretaries. A few practices employed nurses but from the mid-1960s district nurses and health visitors were increasingly 'attached' or seconded to general practices by Local Authorities. By the mid-1970s about 70 per cent of such staff were attached. In the reorganisation of the NHS in 1974 district nurses and health visitors became employees of the Area Health Authority rather than the Local Authority. In 1982 the District Health Authority took over this responsibility.

The so-called organisational revolution in general practice was pioneered by some practices in the 1950s and became widespread in the 1960s. Much of the early work and development was done by the Practice Organisation Committee of the Royal College of General Practitioners. The cost to general practices of employing nurses in practice was greatly reduced in 1966 by the charter for general practice negotiated between the then government and the BMA. This led to the introduction of reimbursement of 70 per cent of the salaries of approved staff to the limit of two full-time staff of each established principal.

The position today is in great contrast to that pertaining when most older practitioners started with a wife/receptionist and a part-time bottle-washer. Now it is common for a partnership of three or more to employ a number of receptionists and a secretary, perhaps a practice nurse and a practice manager. Attachment of nurses and health visitors is the rule rather than the exception.

With the movement of services into the community, closer relationships between community psychiatric nurses and social workers can be foreseen. Within one professional lifetime a one-man band has turned into an orchestra. Unfortunately, the players often scrape and blow without knowing or really caring what their colleagues are doing.

In this chapter we describe briefly the role and the training of different members of the primary health care team. In the following one we suggest ways in which they may be encouraged to work together.

1. The Receptionist

The duties undertaken are based on the reception of messages and of patients as they arrive at the desk. This is the front role, the dragon at the gate. The day may run smoothly, but however efficient the practice no day passes without problems, without difficult questions, without awkward decisions, and not many pass without the potential for some form of complaint or even aggression.

General practitioners have for a long time taken their receptionists for granted, without finding out what responsibilities they shoulder day by day, and have assumed they could cope without training.

In the course of running an appointment system, of answering the telephone, or receiving requests for visits and repeat prescriptions they need the support of practice policies and practice rules. They also need to be able to get on with people, to remain calm and cheerful under pressure, to recognise and cope with emergencies, to possess stability and common sense.

Other duties receptionists undertake may include registration of new patients and temporary residents, pulling records for surgeries and refiling, 'house keeping' within the premises, opening and sorting incoming mail, posting outgoing mail, opening the premises in the morning and closing them at night.

Until recently there have been very few recognised training courses for general practice receptionists. There are signs that this situation is changing.

2. The Secretary

In small practices the receptionist may also function as a secretary, but most large practices employ at least one secretary. Besides audio and typing skills a secretary in general practice needs to possess detailed knowledge of procedures, medical terms, and of the relationships which the practice has with hospitals, the FPC, insurance companies and other organisations with which it does business. She is usually responsible for overseeing various practice systems, particularly those which involve call and recall for preventive procedures. In practices which do not employ a separate finance secretary she may also be responsible for paying bills, calculating PAYE, and for all the financial transactions which are not undertaken by the partners themselves.

In a practice which does not employ a practice manager the secretary is usually the central point of the practice organisation.

A variety of training courses for practice secretaries are available, ranging from extended day release to full-time courses at polytechnics. Advice may be obtained from the Association of Medical Secretaries, Tavistock House South, Tavistock Square, London, WC1 9LN. Reimbursement of 70 % of the cost of providing training for a practice secretary may be claimed by practitioners if the criteria laid down in paragraphs 52.8 and 52.9 of the Red Book are fulfilled.

3. The Practice Manager

The position of practice manager is of relatively recent origin. A combination of factors — the amalgamation of practices to form larger units, the increasingly complicated employment tax and NHS regulations, the growing awareness of many general practitioners of their lack of desire to spend more time in management than in clinical work — has resulted in the creation of a new animal, the practice manager.

In a practice where a practice manager is employed, he or she has delegated responsibility under the direction of the managers for the efficient running of the practice.

The role of the practice manager involves knowledge of all the activities which take place in the practice and responsibility for ensuring that conditions are right for satisfactory performance. He or she will order and maintain all supplies and equipment, will be responsible for the efficient running of all the practice systems, will allocate duties, organise duty rosters and holidays.

The practice manager also acts as the liaison between partners and staff. It is a demanding job. Pre-employment training and in-service training is available. Reimbursement may be obtained under paragraphs 52.8 and 52.9 of the Red Book. Particulars of training and of courses can be obtained from the Association of Health Centre and Practice Administrators, 121 Woodgrange Road, Forest Gate, London E7.

4. The Practice Nurse

In the past decade the number of nurses employed by general practitioners has increased to the point that very few new premises are built without a treatment room in which a practice nurse can work. Many practices working in older premises have adapted a room for the purpose. Chapter 9 contains a detailed description of the role of the practice nurse and the organisation of a treatment room. Many of the tasks commonly undertaken by practice nurses have had scant attention in basic nurse training. It is the general practitioner's responsibility to ensure that his/her practice nurse is trained for the role she undertakes in the practice.

5. Attached Nurses

Nurses employed by the District Health Authority and attached by them to individual practices include State Registered nurses, State Enrolled nurses and auxiliary nurses. Although some nurses work in the treatment rooms of the practices to which they are attached, the majority spend most of their time home visiting. Most of their work is concerned with the elderly and chronic sick (Harris and Jones, 1977). In the care of the severely disabled and of the dying they are the key members of the primary health care team.

For many years the range and responsibility of their work has been underestimated by all but their patients. It has been recognised that they visit to carry out technical procedures, such as taking blood, treating wounds and ulcers, administering enemas and bed baths. It has been known that they provide chronic nursing and support (Jones, 1981). What has not been appreciated by other members of the primary health care team and often by their nursing officer superiors, is the range of their experience and skills.

MacIntosh and Richardson in 1976 published a work study of district nursing. A similar analysis over a period of 3 months in one author's practice showed that, in addition to the nursing procedures she carried out, in 36 per cent of home visits the nurse gave advice on daily living, in 29 per cent she instructed or supervised rehabilitation exercises, and in 26 per cent she counselled concerning personal problems.

In the past such skills have had to be gained through experience. It is as recently as 1983 that the special training needs of community nurses were finally recognised and national regulations and guidelines for district nurse education were put into effect.

6. The Health Visitor

Health visitors are always State Registered Nurses and are usually State Certified Midwives, although some only hold Part I of the SCM Certificate. They also hold in addition the Health Visitors' Certificate of the Council for the Education and Training of Health Visitors. The regulations required of health visitors include statutory responsibilities, i.e. laid down by Act of Parliament. The Health Visitors' Certificate is now obligatory. In Britain there are about 8,000 health visitors, less than half as many as general practitioners. The Department of Health and Social Security recommends one health visitor for 4,500 patients.

Health visitors are employed by Health Authorities, and their management structure is part of that of the nursing profession as a whole. They are immediately responsible to Nursing Officers and through them to Community Nursing Officers and to District Nursing Officers.

The role of the health visitor is:

(1) Home visiting. She is required to visit infants as soon as possible after the midwife ceases to attend. This is usually between 10 and 28 days. Thereafter these visits are made regularly, especially during the first year, until the child attends school.

(2) Clinic duties. Most health visitors are still required to attend health authority clinics which are the successors to the infant wel-

fare clinics. There they have opportunities of advising about child care and feeding and carrying out developmental assessments in association with health authority doctors.

Increasingly these advisory and assessment functions are being taken over by general practice. More and more practices are organising their own well-baby clinics, either shared between the partners, held by one partner on behalf of the practice, or more commonly, each doctor seeing each child registered on his own list.

(3) Control of infectious diseases. Health visitors are concerned with the personal and clinical aspects of infectious diseases and work with general practitioners and when necessary with community physicians to help to prevent the spread of such diseases in the community.

(4) Health education. Every contact between a health visitor and a patient should be an opportunity for health education. Talks on child care and hygiene to groups of mothers, help with health education displays, encouragement to voluntary organisations are examples of her methods.

(5) Social advice. Health visitors function in many practices as a source of information and of the provision of reports, a role very similar in many ways to that of social workers. The health visitor is often the link between many general practices and social work departments of Local Authorities. This role may well change with the growing trend towards the attachment of social workers themselves to general practice.

Three-quarters of all health visitors in Great Britain are now attached to general practitioners.

7. The Midwife

Few practices are large enough to justify the attachment of a full-time midwife, particularly as almost all deliveries now take place in hospital. In cities and larger towns a full-time midwife may be attached to several practices, but in rural areas it is more common to find that one of the nurses attached to a practice is also a midwife and has a double role.

Shared antenatal care with the general practitioner in joint clinics is now the rule. After mother and child are discharged from hospital the midwife makes regular postnatal visits until the 10th to 14th day, when she hands over to the health visitor.

8. Social Workers

Social workers are not often attached to general practice although many are now working primarily in general practice, and a great many more have part-time liaisons of various kinds with a growing number of practices. Most social workers are employed not by the Health Authorities but by Local Authorities through Social Services Departments. A few may be privately sponsored through grants (Forman & Fairbairn, 1968; Paine, 1976). We recommend two books on the subject, Forman & Fairbairn (1968) and Goldberg & Neil (1972), to describe the pros and cons of teamwork with social workers.

The social worker's role can be classified into three parts:

(a) A statutory responsibility based on Acts of Parliament, especially in relation to child care and mental health. The statutory work of the social worker in mental health is described in some sections of the Mental Health Act, e.g. Sections 25, 26 and 29.

(b) Social Services Departments have access to numerous resources, such as grants towards telephone installation and towards adapting houses to meet the needs of the chronically handicapped in the community. They have responsibilities placed on them by the 1970 Disabled Persons Act. In addition, social workers are often able to put patients (whom they call clients) in touch with numerous voluntary organisations or bodies who may be able to provide advice, resources, or support.

(c) The most important of the professional skills of social workers is called 'case work'. This requires an analysis of the client's/patient's personality, his relationship to his family and contacts and particularly the relationship with the professional worker, and then using these to help the client develop insight and the ability to cope with his life. To do this social workers use a counselling relationship with clients, often of a non-directive type.

The essence of counselling is that the individual is offered the opportunity to talk about his problems. The aim is to help the person to help himself. The relationship is non-authoritarian in the sense that it is not intended that the professional should give the client or patient orders, but should be available for long periods of time to share the problems of the client, to listen sympathetically, to probe, challenge and to question, and to work with the client in a sense of partnership to achieve a shared solution to the problems. Advice and access to outside resources is part of the counsellor's contribution, but the whole exercise is designed primarily to promote the autonomy of the individual.

In the past this approach has been distinctive of social workers and represented one of the greatest contributions to the caring professions. Both doctors and nurses have tended to operate on a strictly authoritarian model, although many general practitioners have for years eschewed the notion of 'doctors' orders' and have advocated 'talking with patients and deciding together' (Batten, 1961).

Nowadays general practice, especially through vocational training and its own developing literature, is drawing on the approach of social work. More and more general practitioners are seeking to adopt the counselling method in their own consultations. There is now a society to promote counselling in medicine. The address is 4 Greenland Road, London NW1.

Paine (1976) has described how a group of part-time social workers can function effectively as a social-work team in association with one practice. Numerous other developments are occurring in different parts of the country. The literature on co-operation and collaboration is increasing rapidly (Brook & Temperley, 1976; Graham & Sher, 1976; Ratoff *et al.*, 1974).

9. Remedial Therapists

Remedial-therapists are only rarely members of the general practice team but signs of their inclusion are appearing. Freedman *et al.* (1975), Waters *et al.* (1975), have described working with physiotherapists in general practice and two of us have links with remedial therapists in general practice. Certainly the traditions and skills of these paramedicals seem ideally suited to co-operation and we recommend that opportunities should be sought and taken where available to promote collaboration.

The remedialists can offer an advisory service on rehabilitation, including that for handicapped children, for patients with strokes and for those with disabling disease. The kind of physiotherapy services in the practice described in the two papers recommended above include the mobilisation and rehabilitation of patients in their own homes.

Remedial therapy may emerge as a new combined profession incorporating the separate skills of physiotherapy, occupational therapy and speech therapy. If the benefits of systematic relaxation therapy are confirmed as a treatment for both physical and emotional conditions, remedial therapists could further extend their role. Patel (1976) has reported lowering blood pressure and blood fats by relaxation exercises.

Current Developments

The impetus towards larger numbers of health and social workers serving the same population in the community shows no sign of slackening. The two alternatives for the delivery of care are either that it should be practice based or that it should be geographically based. Although some nursing managers have misgivings, and social services are as yet still organised on a geographical basis, the arguments for continuity of care and increased co-operation strongly favour recognition of a practice population as the unit upon which joint services should be based.

Recognition of this fact has meant that over the past few years an increasing number of professionals have started working from privately owned practice premises as well as from health centres. This raises a number of interesting questions, such as confidentiality, access to records, payment for services (e.g. heat, light, telephone, accommodation) and the possible adverse effects of sheer numbers.

It also becomes more important that practitioners should not only understand the roles and skills of the professionals involved but should also be clear as to the advantages, disadvantages and process of teamwork.

References and Further Reading

Batten, I. James MacKenzie Lecture 1960, *Journal of the Royal College of General Practitioners*, 4 (1961) pp. 5-18.

Brook, A. and Temperley, J. 'Psychotherapist attached to general practice', *Journal of the Royal College of General Practitioners*, 26 (1976) pp. 86-94.

Forman, J.A.S. and Fairburn, E. *Social Casework in General Practice 1968* (London: OUP).

Freedman, O.P. *et al.* 'Physiotherapy in General Practice', *Journal of the Royal College of General Practitioners*, 26 (1975), pp. 587-91.

Goldberg, F.M. and Neil, J.E. *Social Work in General Practice* (London: Allen & Unwin, 1972).
Graham, H. and Shaw, M. 'Social work and general practice', *Journal of the Royal College of General Practitioners,* 26 (1976), pp. 95-105.
Harris, E. and Jones, R.V.H. 'District Nurses. How many in AD 2000', *Nursing Mirror,* 2 (1977), pp. 35-6.
Jones, R.V.H. 'A measure of support', *Nursing Mirror* 153 (1981), No. 13, pp. 30-31.
McIntosh, J.B. and Richardson, I.M. (1976) Scottish Health Services Studies No. 37, 'Work Study of District Nursing Staff', Scottish Home and Health Department.
Paine, T.F. 'Social workers in general practice' *Journal of the Royal College of General Practitioners,* 26 (1976), pp. 695-7.
Patel, C.H. 'Behaviour modification therapy', *Journal of the Royal College of General Practitioners,* 26 (1976), pp. 211-15.
Ratoff, L., Rose, A. and Smith, C. 'Social workers and general practitioners', *Journal of the Royal College of General Practitioners,* 24 (1974), pp. 750-60.
Waters, W.H.R. *et al.* 'Organizing a Physiotherapy service in general practice', *Journal of the Royal College of General Practitioners* (1975) pp. 576-84.

The *Receptionist's Handbook*, published by HMSO for the Department of Health and Social Security in 1981, was prepared by a joint working party of the BMA General Medical Services Committee, the Royal College of General Practitioners and the Association of Medical Secretaries. It describes aspects of a receptionists work clearly and concisely — and is a good introduction for a novice.

Manual of Primary Health Care by Peter Pritchard (2nd ed. 1981, OUP) contains a chapter entitled 'Who is involved in primary care?' and a further chapter on training for primary health care.

4 WORKING TOGETHER: TEAMWORK

Teamwork is not an optional extra or a bit of icing on the general practice cake but an integral part of the whole process. This was recognised in the Alma Alta Declaration in 1978 and was further emphasised in a recent statement by the World Health Organisation. It is our view that effective multidisciplinary teamwork is an essential ingredient of good patient care. But we are aware from experience in our own practices and others that things frequently go wrong. It is worth analysing some aspects of teamwork and looking at the disadvantages before considering common problems and their possible resolution.

Aspects of Teamwork

1. Pooling

Pooling is a form of teamwork in which two or more individuals co-operate in order to share a facility or service. It does not necessarily involve financial partnership and may or may not involve financial exchange. Its aims are primarily economic and administrative. The commonest example of pooling is where two or more professionals share both a building and secretarial services, as occurs when consultants share private rooms or when two or more general practitioners or partnerships share a common building. In the case of general practitioners the group practice allowance is a further inducement to share facilities. Such an arrangement may enable a group to afford equipment or additional staff.

Another example of this kind of working arrangement is the out-of-hours duty rotas operated by most general practitioners in Britain in which practitioners take it in turns to be on call for several colleagues in one or more practices.

2. Delegation

A second aspect of medical teamwork is delegation, whereby someone is trained to perform work which would otherwise be done by the doctor. Delegation becomes cost effective when there is a saving of the doctor's time which, it is assumed, will be used for work which only a doctor can perform. Delegation ceases to be cost effective if the doctor does not make efficient use of the time saved. Delegated work remains the responsibility of the doctor, who has a legal and professional duty to satisfy himself of his staff's competence.

Common examples of this kind of delegation are receiving patients, filing, telephone answering, and some nursing procedures. The assumption is that this is work which the doctor could equally do himself or herself but chooses to delegate.

3. Specialisation of Function (Division of Labour)

The third principle is that the team may include an individual who has a special skill or experience which is not otherwise available to a member of the existing team. When health visitors, for example, were first attached to general practices they brought with them to the teams they joined special experience and skill in advising about child-rearing, in a systematic approach to preventive medicine and in case-finding, which were generally absent from general practice at that time. They retain today in most practices more skill in dealing with feeding and many other child management problems than other members of the team.

Similarly, the secretaries, by bringing specific typing and dictating skills to general practice, raised standards of communication (typed letters and filed carbon copies) which could not be done by many doctors themselves.

However, in general, division of labour becomes economic and efficient only if the individual with the special skills uses them exclusively or for most of his or her time.

4. Discussion Between Colleagues

The most complex and perhaps the most exciting aspect of teamwork is the discussion by colleagues of the problems of their work. The concept of mutual co-operation between colleagues who are prepared to discuss their work and the policies of the team is relatively new. Few so far are prepared to give and take constructive criticism between themselves.

Normally such exchanges will take place only if members of the team feel secure and are on a par with one another. A hierarchy of rank inhibits criticism as inferiors always hesitate to criticise their superiors. Its potential in British general practice is thus at present mainly between partners and colleagues in selected professions, such as health visitors and nurses. The realisation of the concept depends on mutual trust and a genuine willingness to consider new ideas and to adapt policy through constructive criticisms.

Ideally the practice policies which are described elsewhere should emerge from discussions of this kind and should have been well and truly thrashed out in team discussion and be acceptable to all. Similarly the feedback information described in Chapter 5 is a necessary precondition for the review of policies and for the provision of a factual basis for regular discussion. The organisation for such discussion will obviously vary from practice to practice. Many find a weekly working lunch suitable, others prefer evening meetings and yet others prefer group discussion over coffee. The time and the setting matters little; the personal relationships and the willingness to make constructive criticism over the years is the key to progress. One measurement of the success of such relationships is to ask periodically, 'What new service is our team providing for patients which is measurably better than we did this time last year?'

5. The Aim of Teamwork

The aim of teamwork is the formation of a group of individuals who see themselves as working together for the benefit of the patient or patients. A good team allows each individual member to express himself or herself fully, to contribute actively to the formation of policy and decisions about action, to develop sensitive and professional awareness of the strengths and skills of his or her fellow members. Each member is a professional in his or her own right, shares a common code of confidentiality of medical information, is pleased and proud of the organisation in which he and she works.

The Disadvantages of Teamwork

So much is written about teamwork nowadays that it is easy to become complacent about its value. However, like all other systems of organisation and patterns of arrangement, it has its own disadvantages and adverse effects. These need to be considered as the efficiency of every team should be reviewed periodically by the members themselves, who should seek to measure the adverse effects of their own system and do what they can to minimise them.

1. Collusion of Anonymity

Balint, in his classic book *The Doctor, His Patient and the Illness*, introduced the idea of the 'collusion of anonymity', by which he meant that it was sometimes possible for a patient to become lost between different professionals all of whom were apparently dealing with him. This was because no single professional was accepting personal continuing responsibility for the patient.

Such collusion of anonymity easily occurs in practices still and needs to be identified by the members of the team as soon as possible. Having one named partner for each particular patient helps because health visitors, practice nurses and secretaries all know where responsibility lies. Where this is not done it becomes necessary for partners to agree regularly which doctor is accepting final responsibility. At times it is also necessary to agree responsibilities between health visitor colleagues and nurses.

2. Difficulties in Communication

The problems of difficulties in communication are discussed in Chapter 5. Good management must be designed to promote good communications. Lamberts & Riphagen (1975) have given examples of just how complex and difficult it can be to develop teamwork in general practice. It usually takes several years.

3. Time for Meetings

In practices which make a genuine attempt to promote communication and avoid the isolation of the members of the team, regular meetings are always necessary. These meetings may simply be 10 or 15 minute sessions in which two or more people meet together to discuss day-to-day problems and plans, or they may be more formal meetings, such as quarterly staff meetings for all members of the practice team.

The time these meetings take, however, needs to be monitored and assessed because they can take up too much time and may begin to encroach on the time available for patients. For example, in one of our practices the regular timetable each week includes on average two hours with the partners, a further two hours alone with the vocational trainee, an additional 1½ hours per week with the practice manager, the health visitor, the district nurse, and the doctors' secretary. This total of 5½ hours is equivalent, at an average consulting rate of eight patients per hour, to 44 consultations per week. In other words, the time spent each week in discussing the work of the team has been allocated a higher priority than seeing an additional 44 patients.

This problem is further discussed in the next section of this chapter.

Common Problems in Teamwork

1. Problems Based on Method of Employment

Members of the primary health care team who work together in practices consist of three groups:

(a) those who are self-employed, independent contractors: general practitioner principals.
(b) those who are employees of the partnership: receptionists, secretaries, practice nurses, record clerks, practice managers.
(c) those who are seconded to the practice but are employees of another authority: nurses, health visitors, occasionally employees of the social service department.

In a team which is functioning well the basis of employment does not matter. However, in practice it often does, and in the early years especially a conflict of authority and loyalties may be a potent factor in preventing a group of individuals becoming a team.

It is sometimes difficult for general practitioners who have been independent contractors for many years to be aware of the complexities which can arise for field workers like district nurses and health visitors. They carry major clinical responsibilities in the practice, such as in the care of the dying or of ill-treated children, while at the same time they are professionally and legally responsible to a tier of senior nurses who form the nursing administrative hierarchy. The complexity of this relationship is enhanced by the fact that there are usually several grades of senior nurses, for example, nursing officers, senior nursing officers, nursing officer (community services), culminating in the chief nursing officer who is a member of the district management team.

With the best will in the world health visitors and district nurses find themselves facing two ways because they simultaneously have real responsibilities to their professional superiors and yet have a real wish to be active and responsible members of primary health care teams. Instead of decrying the lack of progress of team work in primary health care it is sometimes worth considering how much has been achieved in spite of the difficulties this structure imposes.

The third category of staff, those employed by the practice, have different but equally important relationships. If attached staff have loyalties outside the practice then employed staff by contrast have employer responsibilities within it. Since a good working partnership demands a free and easy sharing of confidences and ideas, and at times honest disagreements, it may be difficult for primary teams to function unless the staff are very secure and relationships are good. Sometimes employed staff are looking over their shoulders, being careful not to offend the doctor who is not just a doctor but also their employer.

Finally, the doctors themselves may be problem members of teams. Having no hierarchical superior and having a long tradition of clinical freedom and autonomy doctors may be reluctant to share decision-taking. They may not listen. They may hold out against suggestions for change sometimes in the face of overwhelming evidence.

It follows that while all members of a team have a personal responsibility to make it work, the doctors have particular responsibility to be sensitive to the position of their colleagues, to go out of their way to listen carefully to the views of others, to give everyone an opportunity to participate, to share policies as much as possible, and to respect others' wishes and feelings. Undoubtedly the development of small group work in vocational training schemes, especially those which emphasise awareness and relationships can be important in sensitising practitioners during their period of vocational training. Understanding of small group interaction can be most helpful when they find themselves working in small group settings in group practices.

2. Teamwork Takes Time

This simple fact is widely overlooked, sometimes ignored and occasionally resented. The fact is that teamwork is one aspect of human relationships. All human relationships are dominated by time.

(a) Meetings Take Time. General practitioners — most of whom are concerned about the booking rate for their consultations with patients — are much less aware that decisions about time for meetings are equally important. Yet the arguments and the issues are the same.

As a general rule meetings of under ten minutes or so dictate the content of the exchange, confining it to the quick exchange of factual information. Ten-minute meetings can be very useful for informing other members of the team about events — Mrs James went into hospital last night — Mrs Smith has had her baby — did you know that Mr X died whilst away on holiday? Short meetings which turn unplanned into long meetings are a recipe for disaster because they will inevitably impinge on the working schedules of the busier members of the team, will create resentments and will soon lead to absent members who will say, probably rightly, that they 'cannot afford the time'.

The time required for meetings must depend upon the nature of the business and its complexity, the number of people involved and the length of time they have known each other.

There is a working rule based on our experience. Meetings between two, three and four people, e.g. health visitor, district nurse, doctor or midwife, can be fruitful on the basis of twenty minutes to thirty minutes once or twice a week. For a difficult topic or where there is known to be confusion or disagreement between members of the team about twice this time should be allocated.

Another useful formula is to have a working lunch precisely between 1 to 2 p.m. in the practice. This can be a very effective way of working without intruding too much on the working week.

(b) Infrequent or Too Frequent Meetings. Practitioners should beware of infrequent meetings called only in moments of crisis. They should also beware of too frequent meetings, which become a bore and a waste of time. It is helpful if the reasons for which the meeting is held are made explicit, whether the meeting occurs on a regular basis or sporadically.

3. Confidentiality

All members of the team should share the same code about confidentiality of information and have a very clear understanding of what this is. Members who cannot accept the code for any reason may have to miss parts of meetings. Getting confidentiality right is an absolute requirement for the team.

One of the subtler difficulties is the requirement for sharing of information between the nursing members of the team and their hierarchy. District nurses and health visitors often have to report to their superiors and all members of the team including the doctor and other members such as practice sisters and practice managers should be aware of this. It should be clear on each occasion how much has been discussed within a team and how much may be going outside the practice. A team's collective loyalty to the patient demands at least this.

4. Conduct of Meetings

(a) Interruptions. Even a good team working in good conditions and meeting regularly can find its work disorganised if one or other member of the team is constantly being interrupted. The commonest interruption in general practice is of course the telephone and difficult conflicts can arise. Doctors, health visitors and nurses will naturally be reluctant to put patients off and yet do not wish to break up a team meeting if they answer the call.

Careful planning can do much to resolve these difficulties. First of all it is helpful to meet at a time when patients do not expect doctors, nurses and health visitors to be available, i.e. meeting in the middle of normal surgery hours is bound to lead to some patient calls. Secondly, many patients can be helped if the staff say that doctor or Miss X is at a meeting but will ring back in, say, half an hour. Thirdly, some interruptions have to be accepted as part of the working reality of the job. It is however important to keep a track of them and not to allow them to become too intrusive or effective teamwork will inevitably suffer.

(b) The Setting. The place where meetings occur is important. Factors such as time and space may dictate the setting but there is much to be said for meetings with district nurses and health visitors taking place in their rooms.

(c) Decisions Yes, Actions No. Short day-to-day meetings between the health visitor and the doctor or health visitor, midwife and doctor may not need any formal documentation and indeed too much paper can be counter-productive. Once however a formal meeting has been called, such as a meeting of all the

doctors and nurses in the practice to review problems and policies, it is necessary to ensure that someone records the decisions because these minutes represent springboards to subsequent action. A named individual should be responsible for seeing that they are put into effect, otherwise important meetings can take place and no results may materialise.

5. Leadership

Leadership of the primary health care team is a complex subject and one which needs careful thought. There is no doubt it can pose a problem.

There has been an enormous amount of research and study into the dynamics of the behaviour of people when they are in a small group in recent years. It has been shown quite clearly that the role of the leader is of special importance. In some of the most important group exercises of all time, notably the Balint studies, the results critically depended upon the leader. In many other settings, for example on vocational training courses, the importance of the leader has been confirmed on a wide scale.

In the interest of clarity it is first necessary to disentangle different concepts of leadership for the very word can mean different things to different people. Some people see leadership as that of a neutral chairman who will facilitate the work of a group. Others see the leader as being responsible for planning and contributing to the direction of group activity. Others see leadership as a kind of supervisory controlling role.

However, working within the team context in practice, the different members of the same team working together in the same building increasingly believe that the contributions of all the professions are approximately equal and that the privileges and responsibilities for leadership should be shared. The position of leader (if indeed there is to be one) should either rotate or at least not to necessarily fall to the doctor. In practice it is not so simple. The position of the different health professionals in society is not the same and is not equal. There are six separate reasons why the doctor is different.

(a) The first of these is that the doctor has legal responsibilities contained in the concept of the 'registered medical practitioner'. He is committed to his terms of service under the National Health Service. Thus if, for example, a team decision were to be that a patient was making unreasonable demands on the practice and was asking for too many home visits, even if the team were unanimous any subsequent complaint by the patient would be directed to the general practitioner personally. He or she would face the Medical Services Committee. He or she would have remuneration withheld if found in breach of the terms of service. Similarly, a clinical error such as failing to diagnose meningitis in a feverish child may lead to an action in the Civil Courts against the doctor for a sum exceeding a third of a million pounds. Such actions are not taken against the other members of the team, and indeed it is almost certain that they are not legally accountable or liable in the same way.

(b) Doctors are members of a relatively well established profession, one which is frequently seen as a model for other professions. The church, law and medicine have always had a special position in society. In a patient's eyes a doctor is seen as someone special and has corresponding responsibilities. The majority of people who come to the practice expect at present either to see the doctor, a colleague or another member of the team working in association with the doctor. Although attitudes are changing, this attitude still remains a potent factor in leadership expectations.

(c) The doctors' privileged role in society is expressed in pay. General practitioners, according to the Review Body on Doctors' and Dentists' Remuneration, are paid within the top one percentile of incomes in British society. They are paid far more highly than any other member of the team. Indeed in some practices the doctors can earn twice as much as some other members of the team do. Pay is an important determinant of status.

(d) The doctors' training is much more elaborate than those of any other member of the primary health care team. Most general practitioners have spent five or six years qualifying as a doctor, and then have worked in hospital for the pre-registration year. In the last decade the majority of new entrants to general practice have undergone vocational training for at least a further three years; some will have done more. It is common now for a young practitioner to have had in total more than 10 years' training before becoming a principal in general practice compared to the four to five years undertaken by community nurses and health visitors. Furthermore, in many vocational training schemes general practitioners will have studied teamwork, small group interaction, and may have had three years' experience of process-orientated group work which gives them a position of immense advantage compared with many health visitors and district nurses, much of whose training at present is still based in larger groups in a classroom setting.

(e) Yet another distinction is one of territory. Although health centres are neutral territory owned by health authorities on which doctors, nurses, midwives, social workers and practice nurses can meet on equal ground, four-fifths of the premises used by British general practitioners are owned by doctors.

(f) Finally there remains one major factor which also effects the nature of the patient/professional relationship — continuity of care. One of the essential features of British general practice is that the general practitioner once appointed tends to stay in the same place long enough to get to know his or her local community very well, and to build up long-term relationships with patients. Although some doctors move, and probably more move nowadays than in the past, it is still common for general practitioners to be twenty or more years in the same practice. Cartwright and Anderson in 1980 found that the average patient from a randomly selected sample had nine years continuity of care with their general practitioner and as many as a third had fifteen years.

By contrast, under the present system of organisation, health visitors, district nurses and midwives tend to work in practices for much shorter periods of time. Because of their career structure, they move frequently and move on for experience or promotion. The effect, however, is that general practitioners have longer relationships with patients than the other members of the health care team, and some general practitioners find that they are now working alongside their third, fourth or fifth health visitor or district nurse. In primary health care work this difference can be critically important. The doctor builds up a greater knowledge about families and their patterns of behaviour, not necessarily because he is any more able or skilled than the health visitor or nurse but simply because he may have worked with the family for ten years longer. This difference between the members of the team is serious and deserves considerable research and thought. It is to be hoped that the nurses involved with primary health care will find ways of adapting their career structure to provide greater continuity of care so that they too can acquire equally long and productive relationships with families.

Given all these factors it is clear that there are a number of pressures all pointing in the same direction — namely to make the doctor the leader of the team. These pressures can be so strong that in many cases the doctor emerges as the team leader almost willy-nilly. This may be welcomed or resented by the doctor concerned, and may be accepted or resented by the other members of the team, according to personalities and circumstances.

Approach to Leadership

The resolution of the problem of leadership is one of the most difficult and sensitive aspects of the whole development of British primary health care. We believe that the following approach to leadership which we have tested in our own practices is reasonable in the early 1980s but should be constantly reviewed and adapted in what is a fast changing situation.

1. Initiatives

First of all we believe that the doctor should accept the responsibility for initiating teamwork if this is not already happening in the practice. By starting with very small meetings often in pairs (e.g. health visitor and doctor or nurse and doctor), issues of leadership are unlikely to emerge. Useful and productive discussions can take place without the problem arising.

When the time comes to initiate group meetings the doctor should initially be prepared to accept the leadership or chairmanship of such meetings with a clear understanding that at the first suitable opportunity chairmanship will be shared or rotated among other members of the team. When in the chair, doctors should use their position to build up the team as a whole and should in particular ensure that the views of all the members of the team are heard, that everybody gets adequate opportunity to participate and to discuss the issues of the day. The doctor should not in our view feel guilty about this leadership issue; he or she is likely in present circumstances to be at least as good a leader as any other and may, for the reasons listed above, be better placed to get things going than others. In the long term team leadership is certainly going to be shared. In the mid-1980s the overriding aim is to get teamwork started at all.

2. Social Activities

An important but little analysed aspect of teamwork is paying appropriate respect to the life events of different members of the team when these occur. Events such as marriage or completing twenty years in the practice, passing an examination, or retirement or leaving are of great significance to the individual person. One simple and very important form of teamwork is for these to be noted and if appropriate celebrated by the team as a whole. All teams need to share social activities as well as working ones, and finding an appropriate 'excuse' to have a drink or go out for a meal together will do as much to make teams work as many a formal meeting. A Christmas party is important and many practices have summer outings when members of the team go off together to see some other organisation or institution. Generous leaving presents (which can be an appropriate practice expense for tax purposes) adds to the feeling among team workers that they are respected as people and that their contribution has been appreciated. Although some of these suggestions lie within the province of the doctors, in a practice which is working well initiation of social activities arises as often from staff as from managers.

3. New Members

The greater the importance of the team the greater the importance of new members joining it. It follows that the selection and introduction of new team members should be carefully thought through.

As far as employed staff are concerned, general practitioners are gradually becoming more professional in the selection process. Vacancies in a practice should as a normal rule be first offered to all existing team members. The responsibility for placing advertisements often rests with the practice manager in conjunction with one or more partners according to the internal responsibility of the partnership. Interviewing for new staff is time consuming but although it sometimes seems laborious it is a particularly important activity. One bad appointment can slow down a team. Two or three can wreck it.

Before any appointment is advertised a written job description should be agreed by the partnership as a whole and this is a major method of improving practice organisations. Defined responsibilities of each new appointment can tidy up and remedy some of the inevitable overlap which exists in any organisation. The job description should always include a sentence stating that new requirements will arise and it will be the responsibility of the job holder to adapt to these in the course of his or her duties. Many practices arrange to have in their contract 'responsible initially to the practice manager and ultimately to the partners as a whole'. All partners should be familiar with the job description and at least one partner should have personal responsibility for writing the contract and signing it on behalf of the partnership as a whole. Employment contracts are considered in more detail in Chapter 12.

Conclusion

Groups and practices develop over the years a group identity or personality of their own. There are happy teams and hectic teams, complaining teams and miserable or aggressive teams. Although the kind of team identity which emerges depends partly on the personalities of individual members a tremendous amount depends on the management ability and insight of the general practitioners. Good team leaders are usually made not born.

References and Further Reading

Balint, M. *The Doctor, His Patient and the Illness,* 2nd ed. (London: Pitman, 1964).

Cartwright, A. and Anderson, R. 'Patients and their doctors', 1977 Occasional Paper 8 (London: Royal College of General Practitioners).

______ *General Practice Revisited* (London: Tavistock Publications, 1981).

Lamberts, H. and Riphagen, F.F. 'The team in primary health care', *Journal of the Royal College of General Practitioners,* 25 (1975), pp. 745-52.

Chapter 4: Section 2: Examples of Teamwork

1. Child Care Surveillance

A plan for parents showing recommended times for appointments for child care surveillance — three-partner practice in Exeter

---

We like all the children in our practice to have a regular series of check-ups and immunisations.

The programme we are following is shown below and is the same or very similar to the programme at the clinics. Please bring your child's record of immunisation if you can.

Please always bring your child when you have each appointment, if for any reason you cannot come please *ALWAYS* let us know so that another child can be given the appointment.

Denis Pereira Gray	Helen Chapman, Health Visitor
Ann Buxton	
Russell Steele	D. Smith, Practice Sister

1. Birth or soon after	Medical examination by doctor
2. Six weeks (usually at the same time as mother's postnatal examination)	Medical examination by doctor
3. Six months	Examination by health visitor. Immunisation by sister (Triple 1 and polio 1)
4. Eight months	Hearing test by health visitor. Immunisation by sister (Triple 2 and polio 2)
5. 1 year birthday check	Medical examination by doctor and health visitor Measles injection by sister
6. Fourteen months	Immunisation by sister (Triple 3 and polio 3)
7. 2 years	Examination by health visitor
8. 3½ years	Medical examination by doctor and examination by health visitor
9. 4½ years	Pre-school immunisation (tetanus/diptheria) by sister
10. 9½ years	Booster immunisation (diptheria/tetanus) by sister
11. 10½ years (girls only)	Immunisation against german measles by sister

The check/immunisation due this time is number 1 2 3 4 5 6 7 8 9 10 11

Your appointment is at............... on...................................

---

2. Care of Schizophrenic Patients in the Community

A written plan of care for practice sisters working in a general-practice treatment room — three-partner practice in Exeter

---

Introduction. Schizophrenia now occurs in about one in a hundred of the population and is often controllable by chemical drugs of the phenothiazine group particularly fluphenazine (Modecate) or flupenthixol (Depixol) which is a slow -release preparation.

Aim. The aim is to maintain the patient at home and out of hospital.

Doses. If starting fluphenazine (Modecate) for the first time the test dose of 0.5ml (25mg per ml) should be given. The effects normally last between 15 and 40 days. Seeing all patients every three weeks is a reasonable regular routine but the patient's own doctor is responsible for deciding the exact frequency.

Prescriptions will be written as:

a) Inj. fluphenazine (Modecate) 25mg every three weeks.
Mitte 10

b) Inj. flupenthixol (Depixol) 20mg every three weeks.
Mitte 10

Precautions. Precautions should be taken about side-effects if key organs like the liver, heart or kidneys are failing. Not to be used in pregnancy.

Side-effects. Side-effects are the anti-cholinergic group and include drowsiness, lethargy, blurred vision, dry mouth, constipation, mild hypotension and Parkinsonian symptoms such as twitching or stiffness of muscles.

Care in the Treatment-room. 1. Ensure that each patient on fluphenazine has a card which never leaves the sister's box. Schizophrenic relapse occurs quickly once treatment is stopped so failure to attend means a follow-up appointment should be sent immediately and attendance is then checked by the sister.

2. Give patients time in the consultation to talk about themselves and look particularly for the classic features of schizophrenia which are:

(a) Muddled thinking.
(b) Funny moods, i.e. too happy or too sad in relation to their situation or just not reacting emotionally.
(c) Unreasonable suspiciousness (paranoia).
(d) Look for side-effects of the drugs especially:
    (i) Odd movements of the tongue.
    (ii) Stiffness or twitching muscles especially the face.
    (iii) Odd movements in general.

3. Ensure patient is seen by their own doctor at least every six months and at the same consultation if any of the above symptoms are present or if the sister just feels something is wrong.

4. Test urine once a year and record.

5. Take blood once a year — usually in the month of their birthday for:
   (a) Liver function
   (b) Blood urea

Procyclidine 5mg (Kemadrin). Procyclidine is used as an anti-Parkinsonian agent and is therefore often used with drugs like fluphenazine (Modecate) to counteract the tendency that these drugs have to produce Parkinsonism.

All doctors in the practice are now trying to reduce the prescriptions for this in order to avoid side-effects from the main drug being masked and will discuss this with any patient who queries the treatment.

5 THE PRINCIPLES OF MANAGEMENT IN THE PRACTICE

> The essential unit of medical practice is the occasion when, in the intimacy of the consulting room or sick room, a person who is ill or believes himself to be ill, seeks the advice of a doctor whom he trusts. This is the consultation and all else in the practice of medicine derives from it (Spence, 1960).

The consultation as defined above has always remained the focus of general practice and the purpose of practice organisation or management is to promote the quality of that consultation so that the maximum benefit is obtained by the patient. This statement of practice management sounds simple, but if this primary aim is not constantly remembered there is always a danger that organisation and management will become an end in itself and develop into a self-perpetuating and increasingly expensive machine.

In Chapters 2 and 12 we stress the fact that general practitioners are independent contractors and are self-employed. We are, therefore, responsible for the organisation of our own partnership or firm equivalent of directors of business.

Medical practice is one of the few situations in our society where major decisions about people's lives are taken regularly. Eimerl & Pearson (1976) have shown that the speed of decision-taking in modern general practice is probably as quick as in any other profession.

Business management is now an established discipline and it is necessary for practitioners as responsible partners to understand the principles of good organisation. Organisation management, therefore, should form part of the training of all future general practitioners.

General Principles

There are several general principles which can be applied to all systems of organisation and management in all general practices.

(1) The decision-making process should be clear and understood.

(2) Appointment of staff should not be made in a haphazard fashion without unanimous agreement among partners.

(3) Practice rules should be absolutely clear to all members of the staff and the reasons for the rules understood.

(4) The organisation should promote individual initiative and experiment by all members of staff.

(5) There should be personal contact between those in authority (the general-practitioner partners) and those who are employed by them.

(6) Delegation should be planned individually in the light of the particular skills of each member of staff.

(7) Meetings should be held frequently enough to prevent difficulties becoming grievances.

(8) Management should initiate and encourage feedback on the working of all practice systems.

(9) Information should be shared.

1. Clarifying the Decision-making Process

By definition the final point of the decision-making process in general practice in Britain is the partnership meeting. Both in law as the employers, and as individuals 'collectively and severally responsible' to the Inland Revenue Authorities, the partners in a group practice are legally and financially responsible for the practice. The partnership meeting is where the buck stops. In law all partners are liable for the sins and omissions of all partners; patients can sue the whole partnership if they choose. This means that the partnership meetings, their organisation, their frequency, their minutes, and the way their decisions are translated into action are crucial in every group practice. The frequency of meetings must be by agreement between partners but normally they should not be less than monthly and arrangements have to be flexible enough for extra meetings to deal with particular problems. The arrangement for partnership meetings is often specified in partnership agreements.

Decisions taken at partnership meetings must be recorded in writing. We find one of the most effective methods is to indicate after each discussion the initials of the partner responsible, e.g. 'It was agreed to explore costs of buying an ECG machine. Action X.' The list of 'actions' forms the 'matters arising' for the agenda of the next meeting. There are several reasons why written records are necessary for partnership meetings:

(1) These are business meetings, at which as shown throughout this book decisions about people (staff) and substantial sums of money are taken. Most partnerships of three partners in Britain have an annual turnover of about £120,000 and bigger groups can easily exceed £200,000 turnover each year. Throughout the world it is good business practice to keep a written record of business meetings and the decisions taken by executives.

(2) Human nature being what it is, decisions tend to get left – often just by inertia. It is usually easier to do nothing rather than something and this may mean that new ideas and policies get perpetually postponed. Older doctors especially tend to defer changes; a decision to postpone is still a decision!

By simply having a written agenda at least each month and by listing as items on the agenda all the decisions reached at the previous meeting, an automatic tightening up of procedure is achieved relatively painlessly. This can be particularly important for new young principals, particularly vocational trainees, who on entering a practice often bring many new and stimulating ideas. It is remarkable how much gets done a few days *before* partnership meetings!

(3) If decisions are not minuted in writing some will be forgotten.

(4) Written minutes remind all the partners that they are working as business partners and will make what is implicit explicit. It will soon become apparent if one partner is being left with all the responsibility.

Partnerships in which there are no written minutes often function with one dominant partner who runs the practice. The 'Managing Director' model may work well for a few years but eventually will lead to the other partner or partners becoming either resentful, dependent, or isolated, all of which we regard as unsatisfactory. New partners need to establish what exactly is partnership business, and what decisions can be delegated to different members of the staff. In time, however, the policy should be clarified not only in the minds of all the partners but also in the minds of all the staff, in terms of the kind of decision to be taken by the partners: policy decisions about appointing partners or staff; policy about clinical management of patients or about organisations or individuals outside the practice; policy on accepting new patients; policy in relation to financial shares, and about financial management, depreciation and expenditure on equipment, maintenance and repairs.

We have mentioned earlier and will discuss again in Chapter 12 the importance of the partnership agreement which controls the broad legal framework within which the practice partnership exists, but regular monthly meetings and above all day-to-day contact between partners build up the human relationship which determine how any group of partners functions as a team. The management principle, however, is that the staff should have a general idea of where the buck stops, how the practice is organised and where and why the main decisions are taken.

Difficulties in Decision-making

One of the most important variables affecting decision-making is the number of people involved. Given the desirability of informing, discussing and always consulting those affected by decisions, the advantage of keeping groups small becomes clear. The complications of achieving decisions without imposing them through a hierarchy of authority, rise geometrically with the number of people. Small is beautiful!

Delays

Similarly, one of the worst aspects of management in big organisations is the delay which so often takes place before an answer, any answer, appears. A good decision may become only a moderate, if not a bad decision, if it is long delayed. Partners should always be conscious of how long it takes for a decision to be acted upon in the practice.

2. Appointing Staff

Appointing members of staff is always important. Everyone in the premises has access to notes and confidential information and in a small group of people working together the personality and the behaviour of one member of a team always affects the others. A chain is no stronger than its weakest link, so the partners must vet every single link in the chain of the team.

We recommend that all partners should normally attend all interviews and should be joined by the practice manager or senior member of staff who will have to work closely with the new person. It is useful to have in the practice a typed list of standard questions to clarify at interview. One example is given in Section 2 of this chapter. Further consideration is given to appointment of staff in Chapter 4.

3. Rules and their Reasons

All families and groups of people need to have their own rules and the bigger the group and the more complicated its task the greater is the need for some set of rules. The general principle of management for general-practitioner partners, however, is quite simple — rules should be as few as possible so that staff are restricted as little as possible. A rule should be introduced only when it is a necessary safeguard to patients. Whenever a rule is introduced, it should always be fully discussed with whoever is involved; above all there is an obligation on those in authority, i.e. the partners, to explain fully and repeatedly the reasons for it. Finally, all important rules should be recorded in writing and should be available to staff who have to operate them.

Examples of rules in operation in some practices may be found in Section 2 at the end of this chapter.

4. Encouraging Staff Initiative

The employer — employee relationship is a great responsibility for the employer. General practitioners are fortunate working in relatively small and enclosed systems. We do not have to face the great problems of authority and hierarchy which occur in other parts of the Health Service and in many other organisations.

It is a useful principle in general practice to avoid a hierarchy of more than three ranks. The organisation of partner/senior secretary/receptionist/or junior secretary is probably as much as is comfortable or necessary. General practice is built up on individual relationships between doctor and patient and this should be the model for organisation as well. Organisation often works best with a single practitioner with a single secretary, but obviously modifications are necessary in big groups.

The doctors must seek to encourage initiative. Ideas and criticisms should always be encouraged, carefully considered, and if possible implemented. If a member of staff proposes a different way of doing something and the partners are uncertain whether the new method offers any real advantage, there is much to be said for allowing the experiment. It will provide a healthy challenge to the inherent conservatism of the practice and will inevitably involve the member of staff actively in the organisation. It will promote interest in the experiment among other members of the staff, which is all to the good. Organisations where the staff never make any suggestions or where such suggestions are never implemented will soon lose the better members of the staff or at least lose their enthusiasm and interest.

Just as the model of the relationship between general practitioner and patient strives towards equality and partnership, so the general-practitioner partner as an employer should strive for a partnership relationship with his staff.

5. *Personal Contact*

Most human beings in most organisations make regular contact with other people. Most of the doctors who work in general practice and most of their staff do their job because they like working with people. Strangely enough, however, the high turnover of patients and the pressures of general practice stress the administrative systems of management to the point that the members of the team may sometimes have little or no time to talk to each other and may find themselves rushing home after evening surgery exchanging only a few words.

In particular, doctors cannot allow the stresses and strains of life to be dealt with by 'taking it out' on whoever happens to be present at the time. Such behaviour by doctors only creates guilt and anger in the staff who in turn may 'take it out' on patients.

It is a general principle of management that a good employer sees his staff as individuals with their particular strengths and weaknesses and gets to know them as individual human beings. There is no substitute for personal contact, such as having time occasionally for a chat or staying to have a cup of coffee when the surgery has finished. If we wish our staff to provide a personal service for patients, we owe it to them to care for them ourselves. As a general rule each member of staff should be entitled to a fixed time in the week to discuss any problems with the partner concerned.

6. *Delegation*

Specialisation of labour is a fundamental principle of modern organisation and the division of labour is one of the principal devices for improving output in organisations. Obvious examples include typing and filing, where it is almost certainly true that most professional secretaries type letters better than most doctors!

Allied to this principle is the theory of delegation. If there is work that can be equally well done by a non-doctor, then it is more efficient for it to be done by a less highly trained person, e.g. filing clerks file the letters, which is more efficient than the doctor doing it himself. This principle holds true as long as the doctor's training is longer than that of the filing clerk and as long as the doctors are more highly paid.

The principle of delegation should not just be thought of in terms of organisation but is equally applicable to clinical work. *The Practice Nurse* published by the Royal College of General Practitioners (*Reports from General Practice, No. 10*) suggested the possible clinical scope of the practice nurse as long as ten years ago. Further discussion on this subject is provided in Chapter 9, and in greater detail in a recently published book by Bolden and Takle.

Delegation, or who does what in a practice team, is discussed in Chapter 4. However, the management principle is that it should be flexible, dynamic, and subject to constant review because the history of medicine shows that what is considered to be a task appropriate for a doctor at one time is often equally generally recognised to be the nurse's work at another.

7. *Regular Meetings*

In addition to individual personal contact, it is a general principle of management that meetings should be held often enough to allow members of the staff of any organisation to express their ideas and feelings in the context of a group with their seniors or employers. In the short hierarchy that is characteristic of general-practice organisation, this means meetings between the partners and the staff. There is no general rule about how often these ought to take place but there are two guiding principles: the staff themselves should choose the frequency and the doctors should fit in with them. The appearance of numerous complaints and grievances usually represents a symptom of inadequate communication and a sign that meetings are too infrequent.

In one of our practices the staff meet the partners once a quarter and the different groups within the practice team, such as the three part-time SRNs, meet the partners about every two months. In addition, there are short fixed weekly meetings of the health visitor, district nurses and the practice manager, in order to deal with day-to-day decisions.

8. Feedback

It is useful to consider practice organisation in terms of system analysis. Practices are living growing groups, capable of developing or regressing. One of the most important management principles is that those who are responsible for decision-making at all levels should be regularly supplied with information about the consequences of their previous decisions. Feedback of factual information about, for example, the list sizes and prescription costs are routine through the NHS in all practices. These rough and ready data supplied to general practitioners through the National Health Service are seriously inadequate as a basis for practice.

Modern general practitioners expect much more detailed and much more regular feedback to partners than this and it is the responsibility of partners themselves to organise systems so that this information is regularly generated as part of the routine day-to-day work of the practice and is not regarded by the staff who do it as an unnecessary and additional chore.

What kind of information is useful? First and foremost the size of the list and the way that it is changing, the total number of patients and the frequency with which they consult, is almost basic information if any rational attempt is to be made to organise an appointment system. Keeping regular accounts of all consultations and visits is the only way to detect developing trends and to compare the practice with the results published by others.

We will describe some simple systems of financial analysis in Chapter 19. The relevant principle here, however, is that only by feeding back information about what is happening and what are the consequences, is it possible to discuss, adapt and improve the financial system. Partners today are entitled to expect regular returns on all the main activities in their practice — not just for themselves, but for all the partners. Similarly, members of staff who run parts of the practice should be supplied with feedback about the results.

9. Sharing Information

Teamwork is discussed in Chapter 4. However, it is already clear that the majority of general practitioners in the United Kingdom in the future are going to work in groups with what is likely to be an increasing number of secretaries, nurses, receptionists, and health visitors.

Communication can be defined as sharing information and making decisions. Most of this chapter so far has been concerned primarily with decision-making. Sharing information is, however, equally important. Failure to share information is probably the greatest weakness in general practice organisation in Britain today.

The problem arises because although the general-practitioner partners automatically discuss between themselves all the important organisational issues by virtue of their partnership, and although the senior practice secretary or practice manager is likely to know most of the news by virtue of her job, there is nevertheless a tendency for other members of the team to be left out. Information is not always shared automatically and one of the tests of a good organisation is to assess the formal ways it may have for sharing information among all those who work in the practice.

Behaviour of the staff can be a symptom of failure. 'Oh, I didn't know that,' particularly if repeated, or worse still, 'Nobody ever tells *me* anything' are comments that give a clear indication to the general-practitioner partners that counter-action is needed and more organised methods must be introduced for sharing information.

Most important is the direct and personal discussion between partners and different members of the team. There is, as has been shown above, no substitute for this. It should be the responsibility moreover of all the partners to do it. However, there is much routine information which tends to be forgotten in such discussion or which may not be directly relevant until later. Responsibility may be allocated to a senior member of the staff, preferably the practice organiser, administrator, or senior secretary, and she should have as part of her work the responsibility of ensuring that other members of the staff are informed of important information which is relevant to the working of the practice.

The practice meetings described above also serve as an opportunity for information to be shared and questions to be asked by all members of the staff. In the context of information-sharing, staff notice-boards are also helpful. In one of our practices we list the workload figures and the changes in frequency of home visits and consultations which are all prepared by one member of the staff, the records clerk, and presented periodically to the partners. By putting the annual returns on the notice board for all members of the staff to see, everybody shares the information generated. Sharing information does not just happen automatically; it is part of the responsibility of management to plan for this to happen regularly.

Changing Systems

The principles of management outlined in this chapter are accepted by all the four authors of this book, and govern the working of our practices. There are, however, many general practices where some or all of these principles are neither accepted nor operated.

We do not believe that management systems, however desirable, can be imposed suddenly. On the whole, general practice has always progressed best by evolution rather than revolution and changes in organisation, however good, are usually best introduced slowly with a great deal of discussion with all the people concerned.

Doctor-Staff Relationships

General practice has already made a huge contribution to medicine by emphasising the tremendous importance of the doctor-patient relationship (Balint, 1964; Browne & Freeling, 1976). General practitioners have shown that this relationship or interaction not only affects the way patients and doctors feel but directly influences the quality of care the patient receives.

The principles of managing staff are directly analogous to the principles of managing patients and each of the sections discussed above has a parallel in the doctor-patient relationship. In summary, it all boils down to liking and trusting staff and treating them as we would like to be treated ourselves.

References

Balint, M. *The Doctor, His Patient and the Illness*, 2nd edition (London: Pitman, 1964).

Browne, K. & Freeling, P. *The Doctor-Patient Relationship*, 2nd edition (London: Longman, 1976).

Eimerl, T. & Pearson, R.J.C. *British Medical Journal*, 2 (1976), pp. 1549-54.

Royal College of General Practitioners. *The Practice Nurse. Reports from General Practice*, No. 10 (London: Royal College of General Practitioners, 1970).

Spence, J. in *The Purpose and Practice of Medicine* (London: OUP, 1960).

Chapter 5: Section 2

Examples of Practice Rules

A Issued as 'Guidelines to Receptionists' by a Four-partner Practice

---

1. Appointments

(a) Book according to individual doctors' later activities (e.g. Visits, Dept., Squash, Deaf School, etc). Doctors to check their columns each morning.
(b) Book in the morning rather than the afternoon or evenings.
(c) Book patients who need to see a doctor *with the doctor* and not with the practice nurse.

2. Visits

(a) Do not argue with the patient. Either accept the visit, with a phone number if possible, or put the call through to the doctor concerned.
(b) Don't phone back or get the patient to do so. Deal with the request on the first telephone call.
(c) Bleep the duty doctor with late visits when they are received.

3. Commitments

All partners will provide advance daily information of their additional commitments, repeat visits, lectures, social engagements, etc., to help you arrange the workload around them; otherwise assume they are available for consultations.

4. Repeat Prescribing

State when prescriptions will be ready in the light of individual doctors' availability to sign them. Generally a 24-hour wait.

5. New Patients

(a) All new patients in the allocation area are to be accepted without question for the doctor on take (i.e. in the week before his weekend on duty), or by a partner if asked for by name.
(b) New patients will only be accepted outside this area if asking for a specific doctor and then *must* be on this side of Exe Bridge and please check with the doctor concerned.

6. Confidentiality

(a) Do not give information to a third party concerning patients.
(b) When patients call for prescriptions *ask* for the address.
(c) Do not discuss patients or practice matters outside the premises.

7. Insurance Medicals

These may be fitted in at times when the partners are available for consultations (i.e. not doing something else). Book with the doctor concerned and take a telephone number.

B Posted as 'Guidelines to Staff' in a Three-partner Practice

1. All requests for visits must be entered in the visiting book with name, address, reason for visit.
2. It is the responsibility of the duty receptionist to ensure that the appropriate doctor is aware of each visit requested. The book entry should be ticked off when the doctor has been informed (and has accepted responsibility).
3. All information about patients is confidential: it should never be disclosed to unauthorised persons.
4. Partners and staff must not discuss patients or practice matters within hearing of other persons either inside or outside the practice.
5. The receptionist on evening duty is responsible for checking:
   that the premises are securely closed
   lights and switches are turned off
   incoming telephone calls are transferred and the appropriate receiver informed.

C Procedure for 'Urgent Calls' as Itemised in a Three-partner Practice

If the secretary/receptionist considers that a call is urgent the following procedure should be followed:

(a) Hold the caller and try to arrange for a doctor to speak with the caller directly.
In the morning try first to contact the patient's own doctor.
After 12 noon contact the duty doctor — failing this any partner may be asked to take the message.

(b) Enter the call in the visit book, preferably in red biro, noting carefully the time the call was received and the time the doctor received the message.

(c) If the patient or family ring again — record the second call as before in red.

(d) If a member of staff is not happy with the way the call is handled, please discuss with the practice manager.

Specimen Job Interview Sheet

Date	Comments
Application for post of	
Name .... Age	
Address	
Married/single	? Husband likely to be promoted or moved
Children.................... Ages	? Dependent. What happens when they are ill?
Present position	
Previous experience	? Relevant? how skilled
	? How much responsibility
Education	? Sheltered/exposed
Qualifications...............................	
Jobs	? Frequent/no changes
Reasons for leaving	
Reasons for applying	? Job satisfaction
	? Money? Convenience
Health record	? Recurrent illness
General appearance/manner	
Salary	? Salary expected
Questions asked	? Overkeen on 'rights'
	? Slap-happy
Availability	? When free to start
References	? Relevant

At the end of the interview the following questions should be able to be answered:

How will he/she fit into the practice?
How will he/she get on with the existing staff?
How will he/she cope with the most unattractive part of the job?
Do I like the person?
Do I respect the person?

Grading: A, B, C, D.

PART THREE:

BUILDINGS

6 PREMISES: GENERAL CONSIDERATIONS

The general practitioner's most important skill may be his use of the consultation, and his most used instrument the pen, but both require somewhere to be exercised. Just as the style of one's practice is very much an individual matter, so also the type of premises often reflects the individualism of the general practitioner. What follows can only be a short description of the range of practice premises generally in use today.

The improvements in the methods of remuneration of family doctors in the 1966 Charter led to the introduction of notional rents, reimbursement of rates, improvement grants and a cost rent scheme designed to help finance new purpose-built premises. The establishment of the General Practice Finance Corporation at the same time provided one source of capital from which general practitioners could borrow to improve or build premises. Widespread improvement in the standard of medical practice premises has resulted.

1. The Basic Practice Unit

There are few general practices nowadays where the accommodation consists only of a waiting room and consulting room. For most doctors the basic practice unit consists of a room for the doctor, a room for the patients, and one for the office staff.

This basic practice accommodation can be extended in various ways, which reflect both the increased complexity of running a modern practice and also the increased range of procedures and services which nowadays are carried out under one roof. Many doctors prefer an examination room separate from their consulting room, whilst others prefer twin consulting/examination rooms with easy communication between them. Treatment rooms in which doctors, nurses or chiropodists may work, rooms for health visitors and speech therapists, and a staff common room are other frequent additions.

Furthermore a teaching practice, or one intending to become a teaching practice, must consider the extra accommodation a trainee practitioner needs. Especially important is a room from which he can consult, and a quiet room or reading room in which he may study.

In a large partnership it may be decided to work as subgroups, in which separate teams of doctors, receptionist, nurse and health visitor look after their own practice of patients. In such cases each subgroup may have its own waiting/reception area. Such a system, when used in large group practices, is said greatly to improve continuity of care while at the same time relieving administration and communication (Forman, 1971).

An understanding of the movement of doctors, staff and patients around the premises is essential to good organisation. If a group of doctors is moving into new purpose-built premises, then it is advisable to study the movement in the old premises to try and get some idea of the needs of the new. Points to consider include — the frequency that corridors are used by more than one person at a time; whether particular areas are used by nurses carrying treatment trays, and if so, whether corridors are wide enough; whether the treatment room is sufficiently central to be used to the maximum by the doctors.

It is nearly always impossible to meet all the ideal requirements for flow within the building. Often the waiting area becomes isolated from the consulting units and the treatment room. If this is the case, then consideration should be given to the provision of small secondary waiting areas nearer to the consulting rooms. For example, the doctor may consult with a patient and then decide that the patient needs to be seen in the treatment room. In such cases, it is very useful to be able to tell the patient to go and wait in the subsidiary waiting area adjoining the treatment room.

2. Rooms

An extended discussion of individual rooms, their uses and design may be found in individual chapters. The following list summarises the major points:

2.1 Reception Area and Waiting Room

This is the hub of any medical centre, where patients and practice meet. The design of this area needs exceptionally careful thought to ensure a combination of efficiency, courtesy and privacy. (See Chapter 7.)

2.2 Office

The office need not, perhaps should not, occupy a central point in the building. Ease of access for doctors and reception staff is of course desirable but so too is the need to ensure a quiet and relatively undisturbed area in which the medical secretaries can work. (See Chapter 8.)

2.3 Consulting Rooms and Examination Rooms

Doctors differ in their attitude to their own consulting room, in regard to whether it should be a room for only talking with patients, or whether examination of the patient should take place there as well. One of the differences between hospital practice and general practice is in the realm of consultation. Many practitioners feel that a non-clinical atmosphere contributes to the success of the consultation. It follows from this that some doctors may wish to separate the clinical examination of the patient from the consultation.

If this is the case, then the facilities for clinical examination need to be physically separate from but adjoining the consultation room. If a doctor wishes to see more than one patient at a time, then the problems of sound proofing make it essential for the consultation room not to have an intercommunicating door. Patients must be led into the corridor and into a separate examination room.

Various compromises on this theme are possible. It might be reasonable to have a consulting room with an examination alcove, and with an adjoining examination room so that the doctor could consult in a non-clinical atmosphere, and yet examine the patient in the clinical confines of the alcove whilst waiting for a further patient to undress in the examination room proper adjoining the consulting room. (See Chapter 10.)

2.4 Treatment Room

A separate treatment room is probably the commonest addition to the basic unit. Its size is determined by the projected workload, the staffing structure of the premises and the duties undertaken by the nurse. Clearly a practice which itself employs practice nurses throughout the day will use the treatment room far more than a practice without a nurse. (See Chapter 9.)

2.5 *Nurses and Health Visitors' Rooms*

All practices which believe in the value of the primary health care team should have an office which can be used by attached nurses and health visitors. The room need not be large, but should be equipped with a desk, cupboards and filing space. Its use should be agreed before occupancy. For example, is it for private use by the nurses and health visitors or may patients be seen there as well? Who can use it, the practice-employed nurses and the attached nursing staff or specified individuals?

Reimbursement of expenses incurred by attached Health Authority Staff while working in doctors' premises may be claimed under certain circumstances. The relevant Health Notice is reproduced in Section 2 of this chapter.

2.6 *Staff Rooms, Common Room and Library*

In practices employing a number of staff, consideration must be given to the provision of a rest room. Sometimes a room which can be used for more than one purpose, such as an interview room, might serve. It is more usual for partners and staff to share a common room. When it works well this room can become an important part of the practice, somewhere where staff, attached staff and doctors can meet, maybe over a cup of coffee. The room may be used for formal meetings or can be where community nurses, doctors and health visitors discuss the problems and management of individual patients. Such a room would be a natural place to keep reference books, other general practice and nursing books and journals, so that they are generally available on common ground. The requirements of a common room are that it should be out of the main stream of the practice but not tucked away down one end of the building so that no one uses it. There should be shelves and cupboards for books, tapes, possibly a television set. It should be possible to make tea and coffee and to wash up afterwards, either within the room or nearby.

2.7 *Pathology and 'Sluice'*

Urinanalysis and simple haematological investigations are often carried out in examination rooms or treatment rooms. Such procedures may be unhygienic. They can hinder the flow of patients. A small room designed in such a way that simple investigations can be carried out and specimens, dressings and dirty gloves can be disposed of, may be justified. Many practitioners find a haemoglobinometer and ESR tubes useful. A centrifuge, microscope and Ames photometer can be included. With foresight an incinerator can be planned within the room.

2.8 Interview Room

Often in a busy centre a small interview room is a useful addition; it can sometimes act as an overflow consultation room, or a consultation room for the health visitor or midwife.

2.9 Teaching Room

Special consideration must be given to the additional accommodation needed for teaching. The cost limits (see Chapter 11) make special allowances for practices where it is intended to undertake clinical teaching. The type of teaching is unspecified and might include both undergraduate training, vocational training and teaching members of professions allied to medicine. They allow the provision of slightly larger consulting rooms and of a room for a trainee practitioner.

3. Communications

The practice has to communicate with the outside world and within its own building.

Telephone Systems

The larger the premises the larger will be the telephone system used. British Telecom can provide a variety of systems ranging from small switchboards with two or three external lines to large automatic exchanges with many external lines and multiple internal extensions. The more complex the system the more necessary it is that staff are specifically trained to its use.

When deciding on which equipment to purchase or rent, telephone arrangements for out of hours calls must be taken into account. The following possibilities may be considered:

(1) External extensions from the practice to partners' houses. The charge for connection varies with distance and there is a quarterly rental. This may be practicable if all partners live near the central surgery.

(2) Interception by British Telecom and re-routing of the call to the duty doctor or organisation.
(3) A subscriber transfer system by which the practice can switch all incoming calls to one of a number of previously determined telephone numbers. Each subscriber on the list can switch calls from his own number to another on the list by using a switch beside his own telephone.
(4) Answering machines. They are available from British Telecom or from private firms. They range in sophistication from a set which automatically provides a fixed answer (usually including an alternative number) through ones which give and receive messages to those which incorporate radio telephones.

A practice must decide which system best suits its arrangements. The doctor should always bear in mind that he has a responsibility to provide 24-hour cover for his patients and he should ensure that the system he uses provides a reasonable and reliable service for them.

Call Systems

A patient has to be informed that the doctor is ready to see him and there are several ways in which this can be done.

(1) *In person.* The doctor may come to the door and call the next patient. This has the personal touch but can be time-consuming and tiring if repeated twenty times during a surgery.
(2) *An intercom system.* There are several systems available. It is a good precaution to invest in the best that the doctor can afford. Some of the cheap ones break down quickly and are so unintelligible as to be useless. The doctor can either call reception on the intercom and ask for the next patient to be sent or speak directly to the waiting room. The disadvantage of the latter is that deaf or elderly patients may mishear instructions or there may be three 'Mrs Smiths' sitting there. Patients prefer to be called personally if this is at all possible, and a good receptionist can be as welcoming as the doctor himself.
(3) *A buzzer or light system.* A simple buzzer and light system can be used. When the doctor presses a switch a light comes on beside the name and a buzzer sounds. The light may be situated in the reception and the staff then send the next patient in or it may be situated in the waiting room. The disadvantage of the latter is that

the patients may not know who is next unless they have also been issued with a numbered disc as they arrived.

(4) The more elaborate methods described in (2) and (3) are almost certainly required if an appointment system is in operation and the reception staff will need to know who has arrived and who is next due to see the doctor. If there is no appointment system then just giving the patient a number as he arrives may be all that is needed to ensure a smooth flow of patients, each one going in to see the doctor as the last one leaves, but it does lack the personal touch.

4. Types of Premises

A growing number of doctors now work from purpose-built premises. These can be provided by the doctors themselves or rented either from an Health Authority (health centre) or a private landlord.

(a) Health Centres

The 1948 NSH Act envisaged the widespread provision of health centres by Local Health Authorities. For many reasons the health centre programme developed slowly, and only within the last ten years has it gained real momentum.

Since the reorganisation of the administrative structure of the NHS in 1982, responsibility for the provision and maintenance of health centres has been taken over by the District Health Authorities (DHSS) which now rent accommodation in health centres to general practitioners.

The concept of a health centre was such that all the community services could be housed under one roof. Needless to say, few health centres provide all these services and the contemporary view is that each health centre should try to meet the needs of the local community.

Consequently, a health centre should provide accommodation for general practitioners and their staff, together with health service workers in associated fields such as community nursing sisters, health visitors and midwives— all those in fact who make up the primary health care team. In addition, space is usually set aside for providing those services which remain the responsibility of the DHA or Local Authority: the school health service, the chiropodist, some family planning clinics, children's clinics, and the child guidance service. In some centres it may be possible to provide facilities for a speech therapist, for an occupational therapist and for a physiotherapist. The closest co-operation of the primary health care team with others working in the community can be achieved if they are all based in the same building.

A good health centre should not be cramped for space. The need for a service in a community may develop and lack of accommodation can thwart its institution. A large room, basically for health education, can be adapted to provide all sorts of additional facilities. Many of these services may be provided independently by the Health Authority. Health centres are others built with separate general practitioner and community health sections.

However, if a general practitioner working in a health centre wishes to run any special clinics, then he is at liberty to do so. Indeed, many family doctors prefer to provide a developmental screening or family planning service as part of their ordinary consultation service, whilst often set aside specific time for such work.

The services which a general practitioner may provide from premises within a health centre are virtually unrestricted, though recently some Health Authorities have attempted to introduce some restrictions which the medical profession has successfully opposed. He has freedom to carry on private practice in conjunction with his NHS practice provided that this represents less than 50 per cent of his total practice income (subject to the usual abatements of reimbursement of rents and salaries of staff, if the private income earned in the health centre exceeds 10 per cent of his NHS income – Red Book para. 51.15).

A previously dispensing practitioner may elect to continue his dispensing service from the health centre and his accommodation would therefore include a dispensary.

It is clearly essential that the doctor thinking of moving into a health centre should be clear as to what his accommodation and staffing needs are likely to be, to discuss these with the Family Practitioner Committee (FPC) and DHA representative and to see that his rental contract covers all of them. Chapter 18 explains how the rental is calculated.

(b) Purpose-built Private Group Centres

Private group centres are usually provided by the general practitioner and his partners with the help of a mortgage. This may be arranged through the General Practice Finance Corporation or through a bank or building society. Less commonly, premises are built by a private landlord (who may or may not be one of the partners) and rented to the group of doctors.

There is no reason why such purpose-built centres should not be at least as comprehensive in accommodation and design as the best health centres. The cost rent scheme (see Chapter 11) means that a doctor or group of doctors can finance all interest charges on a mortgage arranged through the General Practice Finance Corporation, by the notional rent (cost rent) received from the FPC.

(c) Adapted Premises

There will remain a large group of doctors who practise from existing rented or owner-occupied premises. Some of these may have provided medical services for many years. Often, whilst not clinically ideal, they may find favour with both the doctors and the patients for reasons of situation and convenience as well as sentiment. In some cases no reasonable alternative building or site may be available.

In owner-occupied premises the FPC will pay a notional rent which recognises the capital investment of the doctors in the premises. This rent is usually agreed in negotiation with the District Valuer. Where premises are rented, providing the rent is agreed to be 'fair' by the District Valuer, the FPC reimburses the rent. Doctors wishing to improve existing premises may apply for improvement grants of up to 30 per cent of the cost. Fuller details of this scheme are explained in Chapter 11.

Comparison Between Health Centres and Owner-occupied Purpose-built Premises

It is difficult to compare the disadvantages and advantages of the two basic types of general practitioner accommodation. In Section 2 of this chapter the main differences are described. Whether it best suits a practice to own its own premises, to rent them from a partner, a health authority or a private individual, depends very much on the local situation, the practice and individual circumstances. In general the decision has to balance the freedom of the practice which owns its own premises to adapt them to changing circumstances, against the relief from responsibility which is inherent in rented premises.

5. Branch Surgeries

Many practices have branch surgeries. The regulations governing the reimbursement of rent or payment of notional rent apply to branch surgeries as well as main surgeries. Doctors may obtain such payments in respect of all approved premises.

Often branch surgeries result from historical amalgamations of separate practices. They may be seen as providing for the convenience of patients isolated from the main centre of the practice. Some branch surgeries are little more than prescription collection centres, often without proper waiting rooms or the facilities for the examination of patients. Some doctors feel that if such patients are really to benefit from the service of the branch surgery, then it should be no less well equipped and staffed than the central surgery. On the other hand, other doctors feel that half a loaf is better than none at all, and even relatively poorly equipped premises provide a place for consultation which might not otherwise take place.

Branch surgeries cause a duplication of services and complicate administration. The costs of such duplication must be set against possible financial gain from additional patients brought to the practice. In some ways, even if well equipped, branch surgeries are a potential hazard to patients since no one has yet planned a completely safe system which enables patients' records to be kept in more than one place at once (except possibly in those practices where records are computer held — or where patients keep their own written records).

Doctors should attempt to evaluate the need for subsidiary premises and decide whether better care could equally or more efficiently be provided at the main centre. If a change in the policy of the practice towards branch surgeries is contemplated it is essential to discuss this with the Family Practitioner Committee. They will wish to be assured that the service to patients will not suffer before giving their consent to any changes. Local communities will frequently object to the closure of branch surgeries. Difficulties may be minimised if patients are fully informed beforehand about the reasons for the change and the arrangements for alternative care shown to be adequate. One main argument in favour of the continuance of small branch surgeries is the lack of adequate rural transport. Amongst the solutions which have been tried is the provision of a surgery minibus service which brings patients into the main centre where the facilities of properly equipped premises are available.

References and Further Reading

Forman, J.A.S. *Update Plus,* 1 (1971), pp. 265-70.

Practice in Health Centres (BMA, Scottish Office, 1977). This memorandum was prepared by a working group of the Scottish General Medical Services Committee for the guidance of general practitioners contemplating taking up practice in health centres.

Thomson, W.A.R., MD, ed. *The Doctor's Surgery* (The Practitioner Ltd, 1964). Although many of the problems described in this book were those facing general practitioners in the 1960s, the solutions are often still relevant today. It is a particularly valuable guide for practitioners wishing to plan or adapt their premises and organisation.

Chapter 6: Section 2

Comparison between Health Centre and Owner-occupied Practice Premises

	Health centre	Owner-occupied practice centre
1. Capital financing	No problem for doctors. Provided by the Health Authority	Need for long-term financial planning and provision of capital at an early stage in a GP's career
2. Capital appreciation	Nil	Long-term appreciation
3. Running costs	Service charges negotiated annually with Health Authority. Appeal machinery	GP and partners pay their actual running expenses
4. Control of use of building	GP has no control on total use though may influence this through the local administrative structure	GP and partners have total control. They may invite other members of the primary health care team to suggest changes in building use
5. Changes in buildings and services	Negotiated through the Health Authority. Although GPs working in the premises can influence the Authority, the approach to innovations may be rigid and facilities may become outdated	Under direct control of GPs system likely to be more flexible and adaptable to changing needs. (Occasionally an improvement grant may be claimed for capital expenditure on patient or staff facilities.)

6. Withdrawal from the NHS	The doctor would lose his right to practise from the health centre (though he is protected until suitable alternative accommodation is found)	Doctor would lose reimbursements of rent and rates, but not tenure of his premises
7. Employment of staff	Staff may be shared with Health Authority. Appointment may be by joint committee — potentially inflexible, disagreements between the Authority and GPs possible. GP does, however, have the right to employ his own staff	Some staff may be employed by Health Authority but the GP controls the appointment and dismissal of all other staff and directs their work (receptionists, secretaries), practice nurses). More flexibility possible
8. Design	Standard design encouraged	Personal variation encouraged

Extract from Health Notice HN (77) 154 which provides the reference by which practitioners may claim expenses incurred when attached Health Authority staff use their premises

DEPARTMENT OF HEALTH AND SOCIAL SECURITY

To: Area Health Authorities) for action
Family Practitioner Committees)
Regional Health Authorities)
Boards of Governors) for information
Community Health Councils)

October 1977

HEALTH SERVICES MANAGEMENT

PRIMARY HEALTH CARE TEAMS
I EXPENSES INCURRED BY GENERAL MEDICAL PRACTITIONERS
II GP SURGERIES — SURPLUS AHA ACCOMMODATION

SUMMARY

This notice gives the Department's views on the treatment of extra costs incurred by general medical practitioners who have nursing, etc, staff employed by the Area Health Authorities working from their surgeries. Family Practitioner Committees may ask Area Health Authorities for help for general medical practitioners who are having difficulty in finding premises from which to practise.

I EXPENSES INCURRED BY GENERAL MEDICAL PRACTITIONERS

1. Arrangements whereby nursing and other staff employed by AHAs work with General Practitioners and others as members of the primary health care team are of

mutual advantage (as well as beneficial to patients). Where the staff work in premises provided by general medical practitioners, however, extra costs can be incurred by the General Practitioners concerned. For work done by such staff as members of primary health care teams, the doctors both incur extra costs and derive benefits and the costs properly fall to be reimbursed with other practice expenses through fees and allowances.

2. There may however be circumstances in which extra costs arise which are unconnected with the nursing staff's duties as members of a primary care team eg Authority sponsored clinics. Where such costs are capable of being identified and quantified, it is the Department's view that AHAs should meet them as a legitimate charge on their administrative budget. The rent and rates for accommodation used by attached staff will normally be reimbursed to doctors under the Rent and Rates Scheme payment which applies to the whole premises. However, additional costs eg heating, lighting, telephone, internal wear and tear, may arise from the services used in the discharge of duties other than primary health care team work. What costs, if any, it is appropriate for the AHA to reimburse will depend on the individual circumstances and are best decided locally by agreement among those concerned.

3. There is of course no question of AHAs reimbursing extra costs incurred as a result of direct employment by a General Practitioner of nursing staff. As regards health centres, the existing arrangements ensure that practitioners are responsible only for costs appropriate to them.

NB: The claim should be made through the appropriate Family Practitioner Committee. It is usual for a percentage of the expenses incurred by attached health visitors and nurses to be reimbursed, depending on the extent to which they use the practice facilities.

7 RECEPTION: THE 'SHOP FRONT'

The initial impression gained by a patient when he enters his doctor's premises is most important. He or she may base future expectations of the practice on their first impressions and this may affect the process of the consultation. How often does one hear the comment, 'I couldn't get an appointment with my doctor for five days,' or 'His waiting room is cold,' or 'The only reading material is four-year-old copies of *Punch* and *Tatler*!'

With the financial help which general practitioners now obtain for staff, rent, rates and running costs of premises, there is no excuse for the old 'lock up' type surgery with lino on the floor, dreary lines of hard chairs and a doctor who has so few staff that he is constantly interrupted by the telephone during his consultations.

When planning his practice the doctor should pay great attention to his reception area, waiting room and staff as in the long run this will certainly contribute more to his professional reputation in the eyes of most of the patients than any number of medical qualifications.

The Reception Area

When a patient walks into the surgery premises it should be immediately apparent where he should report his arrival. The reception desk should be easily recognised and in practices where the premises are large with several practitioners or groups operating from them should be clearly labelled with the doctor's name. The desk itself should be about three-and-a-half feet high and twelve inches wide so that the patient can lean comfortably on it but not over it. Behind the desk should be a wide shelf on which rests the appointment book.

Often the receptionist will have to ask the patient questions which may be confidential and so attention should be paid to this in the design. Confidentiality can be helped by individual reception booths, well screened from the waiting area.

The noise in the reception area should be kept to a minimum.

Telephones, for example, can be of the trimphone variety and tuned to the soft tone which is less intrusive than the harsh clamour of a bell. If at all possible, secretarial and typing work should be done in a separate office. If not, staff who are involved in filing, typing and general office work appreciate a screen of some sort between themselves and the reception/waiting areas.

The Appointment System

During the last ten years most practices have introduced appointment systems. The reasons for not having them include:

(1) Personal resistance on the part of senior doctors who have always had an open surgery.
(2) Rural areas where surgery attendances have to be geared to infrequent buses and other problems of transport.
(3) Small branch surgeries where small numbers of patients and few or no staff make appointments impracticable.
(4) Failure of an appointment system in practice to serve the needs of patients and doctors. Inability to maintain a flexible system.

However, for the majority of patients and doctors a well-organised appointment system has made life much pleasanter. Some advantages of a well-run appointment system are:

(1) Less waiting for the patients.
(2) The ability to make the full use of consulting rooms throughout the day, particularly when two doctors have to use one room.
(3) The more efficient use of doctor time and the ability to direct the workload to periods of the day when it fits in with his timetable.
(4) Because the patient knows that he will not have a long wait in a crowded room he is more willing to come to surgery with a condition for which otherwise he might request a visit.
(5) The practice nurse can have advance warning of the consultations in which she will be involved during the doctor's surgery (such as repeat pill checks).
(6) If one particular doctor is getting heavily overbooked the

tactful use of an appointment system can be used to direct patients to another doctor who is not so busy, if this is the agreed practice policy.

(7) Urgent consultations and children with infectious illness, such as rubella, can be seen between routine appointments by using a side room and the practice nurse to receive them.

(8) Doctors with appointment systems tend to spend longer with their patients in each consultation.

(9) Less space is required in the waiting room.

(10) Follow-up consultations may be arranged around a doctor's holidays or study leave so that continuity of supervision may be more readily maintained.

Some disadvantages are:

(1) Appointment systems which are overloaded for one reason or another will result in patients being told that they cannot see the doctor for several days. This is unrealistic and is not the fault of the appointment system but of the organisation behind it, which should be flexible enough to deal with extra patient demand as well as unexpected emergencies.

(2) Some patients are incapable of making appointments for one reason or another and prefer to 'drop in'.

(3) Running an appointment system does mean that more staff have to be employed to answer the telephone to make appointments. There is, therefore, an increased expenditure on salaries.

(4) Staff need special training in managing an appointment system.

(5) The elderly and women with large families often find it difficult to organise themselves to fit in with their appointment time.

The Lloyd-Hamol appointment book with loose leaf pages is now in popular use and is very flexible. When the doctor is deciding about his surgery times and appointments a number of factors should be borne in mind:

1. His rate of consultation.
2. The times available for consultation.
3. Other demands upon his room if he is sharing it.
4. Re-booking of patients.

These four factors will now be discussed in detail.

1. The Rate of Consultation

Some doctors take a pride in seeing large numbers of patients in the shortest time possible, but this attitude does not make for the good practice of medicine or patient satisfaction.

Probably a satisfactory rate is about eight patients per hour except in times of unusual and extreme pressure. A booking of six per hour should perhaps be a reasonable target. It is vital that patients contacting the surgery at a reasonably early hour should be able to get an appointment that day, if requested, with the doctor of their choice as often as possible. In determining the priority of the booking, patients should not have to be subjected to 'third degree' by the receptionist. Bad feeling created by the receptionist often carries over into the consultation with the doctor.

Some practices find that a satisfactory method is to book at not less than ten minute intervals up until the day concerned. Spaces may then be left, perhaps two spaces on each hour and half-hour for extra emergency bookings. This system has the advantages of providing space for patients who wish to be seen the same day and also provides a few excess patients who can be seen if someone fails to turn up or is late.

2. Times Available for Consultation

Many doctors adhere rigidly to the old 9-10.30 a.m. and 5-6 p.m. regime. If they do this their appointment system is doomed to failure. The whole essence must be flexibility. If the demand is such then the doctor must be prepared to go on for an extra hour or so at each session. It will certainly be repaid many times over by a decrease in patients requesting visits because they were unable to get an appointment and a decrease in the incidence of late night calls for patients who were stalled by the receptionist until the following day. A suggested time for surgeries would be, therefore, something like 9-11.30 a.m. and 4-6 p.m. depending on local and individual circumstances.

Some doctors still run their afternoon surgeries well on into the evening because they start them far too late. Occasionally a man at work will be unable to get away early but this is becoming increasingly rare and the last few appointments of the day can be kept for just such a situation.

There is still a strong resistance to running afternoon sessions from 2 p.m. but this should be considered if space is at a premium in the premises. Many patients, for example mothers with families, like to come at this time of day.

3. Other Demands on His Room

If a doctor has to share his consulting room with someone else it poses a number of problems. The irritation can be reduced to a minimum by making sure that there is at least half an hour between the last appointment of the first surgery and the first appointment of the following surgery, but we feel that sharing a consulting room is a potent cause of irritation between doctors. In addition, it makes it much more difficult for the room to reflect the personality of either doctor.

4. Re-booking of Patients

One of the main reasons why patients asking for an appointment to see their doctor are told that they cannot have one for several days is because he is fully booked with follow-up cases. Of course many patients will have to be recalled at intervals for all sorts of reasons. However, if one doctor finds himself constantly booked up far ahead compared with his partners then he should reappraise his recall criteria. A doctor should be clear in his own mind why he is asking a patient to return to see him. It may be for reasons concerned with routine surveillance in hypertension, for example; it may be because he is unsure of the diagnosis and wishes to check again or it may be to see that his treatment has worked. New entrants to general practice tend to ask patients to return more often because of their inexperience of the natural history of disease and their lack of confidence in their own ability.

If a patient tells the receptionist that he has to make an appointment for a month ahead, the receptionist should be encouraged to use her discretion about the actual day booked for that appointment. If four weeks to the day is already getting booked up or the doctor has other extra demands on that particular day, then she could make the appointment for one of several days either side of the suggested date. Doctors can greatly help their receptionists by not specifying an exact day but saying, 'Please make an appointment in about a month.'

If all these factors are considered when organising appointments, most systems should run smoothly except for unforeseen occasions, such as an influenza epidemic or the doctor being unexpectedly called away. This brings up the important point of punctuality. If a doctor expects his patients to arrive punctually for their appointments, then he should start his surgery on time. It is no good regularly starting half an hour late and wondering why your appointment system does not work.

From time to time it is worth carrying out a simple check on the system by asking patients at random how long they had to wait (a) for an appointment and (b) in the surgery that day. If the answer to these questions is frequently more than 24 hours or 15 minutes, respectively, then the doctor should review his appointment system.

Further discussion on calculation of individual and total consultation time can be found in Chapter 22.

Failed appointment systems are often due to inflexibility, to underestimation by doctors of the consulting time they need, or to lack of understanding between reception staff and doctors as to how to deal with the patient who insists on seeing the doctor and the doctor who is unwilling to see the patient.

As with any other system the need to spell out the aims and to incorporate feedback into how well these are being achieved is essential to smooth running.

The Medical Records

Medical records are most conveniently stored either in or immediately adjacent to the reception area. They take up a great deal of space. Careful thought must be given to the most appropriate method of storage depending on the area available. The long-awaited arrival of A4 size records seems to be indefinitely delayed but practices which use this size have even more of a storage problem than others with the bulging FP 5/6 envelopes. Storage systems are as follows:

(1) Lateral filing uses shelves to store records. This has the advantage of easy access but care must be taken to avoid using shelves too high or low for the staff to reach them, or a good step-up stool must be provided. Remploy make a lateral file which can be simply adapted from FP 5/6 envelopes to A4 size wallets.

(2) Rotating systems. Several sizes of rotating drum are available taking from 5,000-9,000 record cards. These drums have the advantage of occupying less space in the office. The receptionist can stand and rotate the drum thus avoiding unnecessary movement about the office. It is possible to provide covers for these drums to make them secure.

(3) Metal cabinets with drawers are commonly used. These have the advantage of being robust and can be locked. The disadvantages are that it is possible to tip them over if several top drawers are open simultaneously (unless they are attached to the wall), drawers tend to stick and are heavy for female staff to handle. Individual record cards may be difficult to find if a drawer is tightly packed.

(4) Computer storage systems. Several areas of the country are experimenting with the use of computers in general practice. These systems are expensive in terms of capital expenditure but, once installed, occupy much less space. One sheet of 6 in × 4 in microfiche can hold 200 summarised records.

The Waiting Room

The waiting room or area should be so arranged that reception staff can see and communicate with waiting patients. They should look upon the waiting room as part of 'their' territory and responsibility. The atmosphere in the waiting room, the furniture and fittings, arrangement of chairs and pictures has a marked effect on the relationship between the practice and its patients. Rows of hard chairs facing a reception hatch encourage a queuing and cattle market mentality.

Thought should be given to the comfort and colour as well as the durability of the chairs. Some form of carpeting will reduce noise. Careful consideration is required concerning the display of notices and posters. If they are never changed, are jumbled and disorganised it is unlikely that anyone will read them. Display boards, exhibition units or even overhead projectors can be used to enhance communication. The local Health Education Service will be pleased to help with particular promotions and can often supply expertise and professionally designed displays. If there is a patients organisation within the practice it should have its own display board.

Young mothers and their children form an important group in most practices — and young children can cause havoc in a waiting room. The provision of a children's corner is one method of avoiding this problem. It need not be large, but should be physically separated at least partially from the rest of the room. With a supply of toys and appropriate pictures on the walls it can prove a boon.

Finally if there are focal points of interest within a waiting room, such as an aquarium or a row of household plants, their care should be assigned to a specific member of staff. Dead fish and wilting blooms do not aid patient recovery.

Staff

The staff who are present in the reception area, their attitudes, knowledge and efficiency, are as important, if not more important, than the physical arrangements of the reception area itself. Their relationship with both patients and the doctors with whom they work determines to a large extent whether the practice runs smoothly from day to day or whether it lurches from crisis to crisis. The contracts which general practitioners have with their staff are fully discussed in Chapter 12, the financial arrangements concerning reimbursement and PAYE are described in the chapter on practice expenses (Chapter 18), and the philosophy behind the relationship and 'management' of staff within the practice are considered in Chapter 5.

In our opinion these questions are of prime importance. The success or failure of any organisation depends on the people who run it.

Further Reading

Drury, M. *The Medical Secretary's Handbook*, 4th Edition (London: Baillière Tindall, 1981)

8 THE OFFICE

It is a sign of the speed of change within general practice that a few years ago reference to 'the office' was taken to mean the reception area together with the space behind the reception desk. In this space the records were stored and all the paperwork of the practice was done. Today in many practices, and certainly in purpose-built premises, the office is a separate room or even rooms.

This change is recognised in the Red Book which specifies office/reception/records as parts of the practice unit (Para 51, schedule 1 (1)) and suggests that the space provided for typing and secretarial work should be not less than 1 square metre (10 square feet) per 1,000 patients (Para 56 schedule 1).

Work in the Office

Typing and secretarial work form the basis of the work carried out in the office. Except in large practices most routine practice administration will also be carried out there. The post is opened and sorted. Communications to and from the FPC (e.g. returns and claim forms) are organised. Goods are ordered. Bills are paid. Accounts are sent. Just as the reception desk is the interface between patients and the practice on the human side the office is the practice interface with the world of paper.

In many practices the office also acts as the central point for internal practice administration. Staff collect their cheques from the office. The holiday rota is displayed on a notice board in the office. Staff contracts, finance analysis and other papers relating to different aspects of practice organisation are stored in the office.

Positioning the Office

Whether the office is part of a larger room or whether it is a separate room, in order to perform its functions well it should possess certain characteristics:

(1) Typists and secretaries need to be able to work uninterruptedly and without distraction. The office should logically therefore be separated from the main concourse. It should be situated away from direct contact with patients. Moreover typewriters (and computer printers) generate noise which may irritate or disrupt colleagues doing other work nearby unless the office is separate.

(2) As the office in many practices is the central point of internal practice organisation it should be accessible to all staff. From the office the senior secretary or practice manager should be able to remain in contact with and keep an eye on everyday routines.

The conflict between these two aspects may be resolved by separating the two functions either in space (by having two rooms or areas) or in time (by arranging that typing and secretarial work takes place mainly at times when the office is not being used for administration purposes).

Office Furniture

As well as being reasonably soundproof thought should be given to reducing noise within the office. A carpet, curtains and wall coverings all help to absorb sound and make the office more pleasant to work in.

Good general lighting is essential, supplemented by spotlighting or anglepoise lamps where necessary. Desks should have enough surface space for a secretary to be able to work and remain uncluttered. There should be enough storage space in the desk for her to have everything conveniently to hand. Office chairs should be designed for the job rather than converted school chairs or bar stools.

Furniture for the office includes cupboards for the storage of stationery, and filing cabinets for all the papers involved with practice organisation. There is a large variety of filing systems. Filing cabinets come in different shapes and sizes, in single and double rows. They may be fixed or mobile. Files may be roll-out or suspended laterally. Units may be freestanding or flat on the wall, rotating or fixed.

When practitioners are considering purchase of a filing system we suggest that as well as looking in local office equipment shops and writing to the Central Information Service for guidance, they ask colleagues and visit neighbouring practices to see systems in action.

Furniture also includes books. A dictionary of medical terms and other appropriate reference books should be available and accessible to all who use the office.

Office Equipment

The electronic age is advancing. While most practices still use manual typewriters an increasing number now have electric machines. Moreover, it is increasingly common to find dictating machines in use – enabling an audio typist to work independently of 'doctor time'. The advent of photocopiers and word processors in general business use will, we believe, slowly spread into general practice. It is probable that:

(1) More electric points will be needed in offices in order to prevent trailing cables or multiple plug adaptors. To provide in advance for this when it is difficult to foretell where they will be needed, one possibility is to chase an empty channel round the room in the plaster at a fixed height (say 18 inches or at desk height), so that at any time in the future a point can be fixed where needed with little trouble. This work can be done with little disruption at a convenient time such as when other alterations are being carried out or the room is being redecorated.
(2) Space in the office will in the future be at a premium. Many offices are already too small for comfort. Careful planning and adequate office space will have to become a higher priority if the office of the future is to work efficiently.
(3) Practitioners and practice managers will become involved in service and maintenance contracts for equipment to a much greater extent than they are at present. Early delegation of this responsibility to one person will enable them to develop useful expertise.

In addition to normal secretarial equipment and typewriters, if a practice runs an age sex register or other registers and work books, the most convenient place for them to be kept may be the office. In all probability it will be in the office that analyses will be carried out, that prevention procedures will be planned, and from the office that recall letters will be sent out. We judge that as information systems become more widespread the pressure on office space will increase still further.

Tailpiece

When asked what their priorities are most secretaries have replied, 'a desk of my own, some soundproofing, a large notice board — and a desk of my own.'

9 THE PRACTICE NURSE AND THE TREATMENT ROOM

Introduction

The value of having an experienced and well qualified nurse working on the practice premises is now established. Equally important is that the premises should have a treatment room where she can work effectively. Practice premises designed in the last decade have usually incorporated a treatment room and it would be extremely foolish for a practice to build premises in the 1980s without regard to the role of a practice nurse and provision of a suitable place for her to work.

The Practice Nurse

The past ten years has seen a dramatic increase in the number of nurses employed by general practitioners and working in their practices. When community nurses were first attached to primary health care teams in the late 1960s it was expected that they would carry the overall nursing load of the practice. However, it rapidly became clear that this would not happen for a number of reasons. Some community nurses do spend an hour or so a day working in the practice premises, particularly in rural areas. However, the tasks which they undertake are usually traditional nursing ones such as dressings or injections and they are under the control of a nursing hierarchy which may limit the number of activities which they can perform. In addition they have heavy commitments visiting patients in the community, which often preclude them from spending much time in the practice.

For these reasons doctors began to employ their own nurses to work on the premises and often extended their role beyond the traditional nursing duties. It is difficult to estimate how many nurses are now employed in this way, but the number must be well over 5,000. There seems to be a greater number employed by practices in the south of England than in the north.

In this chapter the term 'practice nurse' will refer to those nurses employed by the doctors and working with them in the treatment room. They will be assumed to be trained to the level of State Registered Nurse, although occasionally State Enrolled Nurses are employed in this capacity. If they are SENs then attention has to be given to their roles and limitations of responsibility for medico-legal purposes.

Training

Studies have shown that the majority of practice nurses are women in their middle years returning to work after bringing up a family. Indeed this combination of maturity of outlook and practical family experience is of inestimable value in much of the work performed by the practice nurse.

Some nurses will have added midwifery experience to their basic nursing qualifications but undoubtedly the postgraduate qualification of most value to the practice is that of being fully qualified to undertake family planning responsibilities, holding the FPA Certificate. So much practice work concerns contraception that to have a skilled nurse able to counsel patients, to fit caps and assist with IUCDs, saves doctor time and also has the added advantage of female participation in this delicate area if all the doctors in the practice are male.

The lack of formal training of practice nurses has concerned the Royal College of Nursing, the Royal College of General Practitioners and the British Medical Association for several years and a working party was set up by these bodies to look at ways of establishing a recognised training for this group. The report of the working party will be published this year (1984) and should go some way towards formal recognition of the important part that practice nurses have to play in patient care.

At present the only training available is what the nurse gets in the practice from the doctors and her colleagues, together with the occasional opportunity to go on one-day symposia or short courses designed to meet some of their professional needs.

The Role of the Practice Nurse

Mention has already been made of the diversity of tasks undertaken by nurses working in the treatment room. Of course, the final decision as to what she should or should not do must lie with the doctors, but far too often it would seem that the nurse is left to decide for herself when she has reached the limit of her professional expertise. This will depend upon her personality, training and experience, but it is important for many reasons, not least the medico-legal ones, that the doctors and the nurses working together in the practice must decide guidelines for patient management in all those areas that are not clearly recognised as purely nursing and covered by her basic training.

These areas would include such activities as syringing ears, giving immunisations — including the contraindications — and seeing patients without an appointment to decide if they can be managed by the nurse alone or whether referral to the doctor is necessary.

The role can be as narrow or wide as the doctors and nurses decide and it is this variety of work that seems to be attractive to the nurses who take these posts. Areas which might be included are:

(1) Standard nursing duties, e.g. dressings and routine injections.
(2) Preventive care, e.g. immunisations, screening clinics, routine BP checks.
(3) Emergency medical care, e.g. collapse, first aid.
(4) Use of special equipment, e.g. ECG, vitallograph.
(5) Contraceptive advice and family planning.
(6) Counselling patients.
(7) Special clinics, e.g. obesity, diabetic or support groups.
(8) Assisting other members of the primary health care team, e.g. health visitors or midwives.

Medico-legal Implications

It is important that the doctor and the practice nurse both realise the legal obligations placed upon them. There are two types of liability affecting the practice nurse: her professional liability as a nurse treating patients and secondly her liabilities and those of the doctors as employee and employers, respectively.

The disciplinary structure of the nursing profession changed in 1983 and is now administered by the United Kingdom Council for Nursing, Midwifery and Health Visiting (UKCC), replacing the old General Nursing Council. The UKCC has issued a number of professional conduct guidelines with which all nurses should be familiar.

In addition, the work of the practice nurse involves grey areas where guidelines are not necessarily available and it is important that these areas, such as 'vetting' patients who may or may not then see a doctor, are fully discussed in the practice.

As a general rule a nurse will be liable, under her own professional ethics, for any activity which is clearly a nursing responsibility and for which she has been formally trained, for example, giving routine injections. Any other activities which she undertakes will be accepted provided that clearly defined training has been given by the doctor/employer or some other responsible body. If she undertakes a responsibility or makes an incorrect decision upon a matter for which she has not had adequate training, then there is no defence in law.

The issues are complex and some are still being argued about, for example whether a practice nurse should or should not give a routine immunisation to a practice patient if a specific prescription and instruction have not been issued.

What is clear is that neither doctor nor nurse can evade their legal liabilities and that the professional indemnity for the nurse will be much greater if she is a member of the Royal College of Nursing. Whether she is a member or not, no practice should employ a nurse without adequate professional liability cover, which can be issued through various insurance companies besides the RCN.

Treatment Room Design

There are now many examples of treatment rooms in new premises up and down the country. Anyone contemplating building a surgery should go and see as many other designs as possible in operations as this is the only truly effective way to see whether the ideas of the architect actually work in practice. Never make the mistake of assuming that the architect necessarily knows best where specific design features are concerned. The safest guarantee is to find a colleague who has built new premises fairly recently and is pleased with them and then approach his architect to see if he would work for you.

There are a number of basic principles which should be applied in designing a treatment room and these include:

(1) The room should be light and airy with a pleasant relaxing décor and avoidance of a too clinical or hospital outpatient impression.
(2) There should be plenty of formica covered work surfaces.
(3) There should be more than adequate storage space in the form of large and small cupboards and containers for specimen bottles, syringes and suchlike.
(4) The nurse needs a small office in which to do her paperwork, conduct private and confidential interviews or undertake counselling. Few treatment rooms actually incorporate an office in their design and this will be important as the role of the nurse expands.
(5) A number of working cubicles, either curtained or with solid walls, are desirable. The advantage of curtains are that they allow for a variety of uses. Their disadvantage is that they are not very private. The cubicles should contain a couch and chairs.
(6) There should be a clearly identified waiting area for the practice nurse. This may be part of the main waiting area or a sub-section but it avoids patients waiting for nurse being confused with those waiting for the doctor and also enables the nurse to see who is waiting for her.
(7) Practices are increasing the number of extra pieces of equipment required, such as ECG machines, vitallographs and blood sugar monitors. While few of these extras are bulky they do need to be accommodated and the nurse needs to know how the use them.
(8) It is useful to have a toilet adjacent to the treatment room with a small hatch giving access. In this way the collection of MSUs can be supervised and the patients can be spared the embarrassment of carrying containers through the waiting area.
(9) Any operating table should be able to double as an ordinary couch and should not be an imposing fixture in a small room which limits the activities which can be performed there. Similarly, couches suitable for fitting IUCDs need to be accommodated either in the treatment room or one of the examination rooms.

(10) While a lot of existing treatment rooms have water sterilisers for equipment the modern trend is towards the 'Little Sister' autoclave which guarantees sterility and avoids the risk of short cuts with consequent wound infection. In addition, the supplies of materials from central hospital sources has reduced considerably the problems of sterilisation.

Equipment

All the equipment in the treatment room will be the responsibility of the practice nurse. She will need to check that equipment is functioning properly and to ensure that the emergency trays (see Section 2) are fully equipped. She will need to reorder stocks as they get low.

It is impossible to give a list of equipment to suit all practices, but the following categories are suggested upon which individual variations can be based.

1. Furniture and linen: couches, chairs, instrument trolley, desk, anglepoise lights, sheets, towels.
2. Diagnostic equipment: scales, height measure, sphygmomanometer (desk/wall), auroscope, stethoscope, vaginal speculae, proctoscope, nasal speculae.
3. Instruments for minor surgery.
4. Dressings and applications for wounds and ulcers.
5. Disposable items: gloves, spatulae, syringes.
6. Specialised equipment: Peak flow meter, ECG machine, cautery, electronic blood sugar estimator, haemoglobinometer, microscope, ear syringe, tonometer.
7. Emergency trays: collapse trays, laryngeal tray, eye tray.

The Future

The number of nurses employed in practices is growing. Although there are great differences in the work they undertake definition of their role is becoming clearer. Moves are afoot to establish recognised training to meet their particular needs. We believe that it is important to work towards a system where a treatment room sister is available to patients at the same time as a doctor is holding a surgery. Whether or not the sister should be directly accessible to patients is a matter for each practice to decide, but there is no doubt such a facility has in many practices proved welcome to both patients and doctors.

We still believe, as stated in previous editions, that in addition to providing an added resource and service to patients the treatment room should pay its way.

References and Further Reading

Bolden, K.J. and Takle, B. *Practice Nurse Handbook* (Oxford: Blackwell Scientific Publications, 1984).

Reedy, B.L.E.C. 'The Health Team', in *Trends in General Practice,* J. Fry (ed.), 2nd edn. 1979. *Royal College of General Practitioners and British Medical Journal,* London.

Waters, W.H.R., Sanderman, J.M. and Lunn, J.E. 'A four year prospective study of the work of a practice nurse in the treatment room of a South Yorkshire practice', *British Medical Journal, 280* (1980), pp. 87-9.

Chapter 9: Section 2

Emergency Trays

When a patient collapses it is no use having to rush around trying to find the necessary drugs and equipment to resuscitate him or her. It is best to have appropriate trays already prepared and they might be as follows:

Collapse Tray

Brook airway and ordinary airways
Mouth gag
Tongue forceps
Injection Hydrocortisone 100 mg for IV or IM injection
Injection Aminophylline 250 mg in 10 ml
Injection Dextrose 50% in 25 ml for IV use
Injection Adrenaline 1/1000 in 1 ml for IM use
Injection Prochlorperazine 12.5 mg in 1 ml
Injection Atropine Sulphate 600 in 1 ml
Injection Terbutaline 0.5 mg in 1 ml
Injection Diazepam 10 mg in 2 ml
Injection Frusemide 20 mg in 2 ml
Injection Salbutamol 0.5 mg in 1 ml
Tab Chlorpheniramine 4 mg
Tab Diazepam 2 mg and 5 mg

Laryngeal Tray

Xylocaine throat spray
Laryngeal mirror
Head mirror and strap
Methylated spirit lamp
Matches
Nazal forceps
Spatulae
Swabs

Eye Tray

Sterile minims of:
- Florescein 1%
- Sodim Chloride 0.9%
- Chloramphenicol
- Amethocaine 1%
- Mydrilate 0.5%
- Atropine Sulphate 1%
- Castor oil
- Eye pads and tape

---

10 THE CONSULTING ROOM

General

Most general practitioners will spend 700-800 hours each year in consultation with patients in their consulting rooms. In addition they probably spend a further 200-300 hours at their desks writing, dictating, telephoning or talking with colleagues and staff. 1,000 hours a year is a lot of time to spend in one room. It warrants careful consideration of the design, décor and furnishing to ensure it is best suited to the work to be done in it and the needs of the individual doctor and his patients.

Some consulting rooms are shared by more than one doctor. In such situations the arrangements must clearly be the best compromise possible to suit all users.

Work Done in the Consulting Room

Below is a list of the actual tasks a doctor undertakes in his consulting room. Of these consultation with patients and their relatives, examination of patients and occasional collection of specimens for laboratory investigation are the commonest, the other duties follow as a consequence of these.

(1) Consultations with patients and their relatives.
(2) Examination of patients.
(3) Collection of specimens for laboratory investigation.
(4) Discussions with colleagues, other members of the primary care team and staff.
(5) Tutorials with trainees/medical students/others.
(6) Dealing with correspondence.
(7) Completing repeat prescriptions.
(8) Writing up patients' notes.
(9) Dictating/writing referral letters.
(10) Receiving and making telephone calls.
(11) Professional reading.

Desirable Features

So much of the work which has to be done involves sitting, talking with people, writing and reading. Relatively little involves much moving about.

The ideal room must be designed with these needs in mind. It must have good sound qualities, that is external noise should not intrude and conversations in the room should not be overheard outside. The seats need to be comfortable and easily manoeuvrable. Some doctors will wish to have a swivel armchair for themselves or for their patients; others prefer armchairs. A large beanbag may be a useful feature as well as providing an ideal soft examination couch for small children.

The desk on which the telephone and records will rest and writing be done also needs special consideration. It should not intrude on the general atmosphere of the room and it is doubtful if it should be placed like a barrier between doctor and patients. Most doctors use their desk as a side table on which to place these things, turning to the desk to write when necessary.

A desk with good drawer space enables paper, forms and other equipment to be stored away to avoid a cluttered appearance.

Much of the time a doctor spends in his room he will need artificial light. Good light fittings can enhance the relaxed atmosphere of the consulting room, especially when coupled with properly-thought-out décor of carpets, curtains and wall decoration. The homely touch and family pictures and toys for small children completes the scene.

Unfortunately, this pleasant domestic setting requires some clinical components as well. Perhaps an examination couch in an alcove separated by either a screen or curtains. In addition, most doctors will want to have a wash basin unit and small cupboard for instruments in their consulting room as well as in the examination room. Some of the vanitory units currently available fit better with the décor of the consulting room than the plain white washbasin and stainless steel instrument cupboard.

The choice of furnishing and fixtures is enormous. Doctors should explore ideas in colleagues' premises as well as spend time looking around furniture stores. It might be useful to consult a professional interior designer or at the very least an interested female member of staff. Better still, most married male doctors should ask their wives' advice.

Where To Get Things

Apart from the modern furniture super stores, modern equipment is described in many of the weekly medical journals, some of which now feature a regular best buy series. Most of the major national medical meetings now run parallel equipment exhibitions. For doctors contemplating the expenditure of thousands of pounds a visit to such an exhibition may well prove both worthwhile and fun.

Whose Territory?

Practitioners are seldom aware quite how much their personality is expressed in their consulting rooms. Pictures and prints indicate hobbies and interests. Furniture and its position express attitudes to people and to the consultation. Colours and fabrics can reflect austerity or warmth.

Each consulting room is stamped with the personality of the doctor who uses it. This has the effect of more firmly defining it as his or her territory. General practitioners should, we believe, be aware of the intimidating or welcoming affect their rooms may have on patients.

11 PREMISES: PLANNING AND IMPROVING

Few general practitioners are practising in premises which have remained unchanged over the past twenty years. The changes may have been relatively minor, or have involved major upheavals or a move to new premises. We believe that practitioners are becoming more aware of deficiencies in their premises and methods of working — and that most general practitioners will at some time be involved in the financing and design of improvements or premises which is the subject of this chapter.

1. Planning Purpose-built Premises

Although most doctors who join existing practices will not be involved in planning new premises, all doctors should be aware of certain basic considerations in the planning of purpose-built premises and an understanding of them will help the prospective partner assess the premises from which he may be working.

Architects can give tremendous help to doctors designing premises, but they need help themselves in understanding their clients' requirements. It is important to prepare a clear written brief, in which the doctors list their needs, state reasons for them and indicate priorities. The preparation of such a document by the partners will take time, but should help them in thinking through the new pattern of work which the new building may encourage. When a new element in primary care is to be introduced, for example a treatment room when the doctors did not have one before, then the architect should know in what way the existing work pattern of the doctors is expected to change in the new building.

A second consideration is that everyone who expects to work in the new building should be involved in the planning from an early stage. Receptionists, secretaries, nurses, health visitors and practitioners have different requirements and different priorities. Early consultation will help minimise mistakes in design which may be costly or impossible to correct after the building is completed.

Advice is available from various sources. The Central Information

Service for General Practice is an advisory service which is available to all general practitioners in the United Kingdom. Its secretary may be contacted at the Royal College of General Practitioners' headquarters. It has published a gazetteer of general practice which contains much practical advice. Visits to other practices, sometimes with staff or architect, are also extremely valuable as a way of crystallising ideas. Design points which are successful may be incorporated, unsuccessful design avoided.

(a) Health Centres: Special Points of Design and Financing

When a health centre is planned, all the general practitioners practising in the immediate area have a right to move into the new centre. Often the initiative in starting the process of designing and building a health centre comes from some of the local general practitioners themselves. At an early stage, all general practitioners in the area are notified of the intention to plan a health centre and are offered the use of its facilities. If a majority indicate support for a health centre then the project takes a step forward.

All those interested should have an opportunity of taking part in the planning decisions, and at least one of the general practitioners concerned will be appointed to the project planning committee. Thus, the general practitioners who will work in the building can have an important say in the design of the building. The more interest the doctors take in the planning the better the building is likely to be.

In large health centres there will almost certainly be health or local authority staff working in their own sections. For example, the senior nursing officer and the district community physician may have their offices there, and they themselves may have secretarial and administrative assistants. The district social services team may also be based in the same building. Such a centre increases the general practitioner's chances of meeting those working in other fields of community care and should be valued as an opportunity to reduce sectional barriers and improve the quality of care available to patients.

The doctor is expected to provide all his own practice equipment, whilst the authority will provide the standard fixtures. There can be a lot of disagreement over what is considered standard and what is extra. Equipment such as an electrocardiograph might be considered an extraordinary item, whereas wall-mounted sphygmomanometers might be standard. The DHA may agree to provide extra equipment and charge the doctor an annual fee for its lease.

There is another category of equipment which includes items which are shared. For example, if a treatment room is used by the DHA Family Planning Clinic, then the provision of sterilisers and even specula might be considered as for joint use. In the same way, an audiometer would usually be needed for child developmental clinics but the DHA might agree that such items could be used by the general practitioners. There is no set rule about charges in these circumstances. They should be negotiated individually.

The payment which a general practitioner makes to the Health Authority for use of health centre premises consists of two elements. The first is rental for the premises themselves which is reimbursed. The second is a consolidated service charge (further discussed in Chapter 18). The service charges are deducted by the FPC from the quarterly payments made to practitioners. They constitute a business expense and should be charged against tax. Although rent reimbursement in most health centre practices is a book transaction at FPC level, it is essential for the correct calculation of practice expenses that the rent be declared as a practice expense in the practice accounts (see Chapter 18: Section 2.)

(b) Private Purpose-build Centres: Special Points of Design and Financing

The same basic considerations of design apply equally to private purpose-built premises and health centres. In the former, the doctor is very much more involved for not only will he practise from the premises, but over the course of years he will become the owner of the freehold property. As such the building may more readily reflect the personalities of those working in it.

Many private purpose-built centres are financed by doctors, through a loan from the General Practice Finance Corporation. This is a government guaranteed body which raises money on the normal City of London money market. Consequently it varies its interest rate from time to time according to the standard market forces in operation at that moment. Loans are usually granted for a fixed term at a fixed rate of interest. However from November 1982 practitioners have had the option of borrowing at a variable rate as an alternative to a fixed rate.

Under the cost rent scheme, summarised in Section 2 of this chapter, the appropriate Family Practitioner Committee pays doctors who build approved 'purpose-built' centres a 'cost rent' which is related to the interest charged by the GPFC for the loan. This means that most doctors who partake in this scheme have to repay the capital involved in the building but in effect receive an interest-free loan. There are however several points of practical importance.

(i) The effective rate for cost rent purposes is that rate of interest being charged at the time the doctor accepts a tender from a builder for the new purpose-built building, but the rate of interest charged by the Finance Corporation is that rate of interest currently in force at the time the doctor draws his first tranche of the loan. For example: if the loan is being sought at a time of rapidly varying money supply, rates of interest might change within months and the doctor could find himself with a fixed cost rent at, say, 16 per cent but an interest rate being charged by the Finance Corporation at, say, 17 per cent. (If he were fortunate, of course, interest rates might move in the opposite direction and he might find his cost rent being paid at a slightly higher rate than he was being charged on his loan.)

It is therefore important that solicitors and accountants involved in the arrangement of such a loan should be aware of these problems and wherever possible try to negotiate the acceptance of the tender and the drawing of the first tranche from the Finance Corporation at one and the same time. It is surprising how difficult it is to make such a coordinated arrangement, but most banks are prepared to make a bridging loan to doctors to meet initial expenses to allow the drawing of the first part of mortgage to coincide with the acceptance of a builder's tender.

(ii) Another common problem which requires doctors to borrow money before they are ready to draw a mortgage from the General Practice Finance Corporation is that land purchase often precedes the acceptance of a builder's tender by many months. The security of the land is usually sufficient to guarantee a bank loan. If bank managers are not prepared to meet the doctors' loan requirements against such a security, other short-term loans might be raised by the doctors themselves through insurance companies. It is important to gain the Family Practitioner Committee's approval at the earliest possible stage to ensure that all allowable expenses may be claimed later.

(iii) It is important to ensure that the Regional Medical Officer of the DHSS gives his approval to the design of the proposed premises. The design must meet the basic requirements laid down in the regulations concerning the cost rent scheme. If doctors build premises which do not meet those requirements, they may find that their cost rental will be affected. There are, incidentally, cost limits which are reviewed at regular intervals, but in a time of rapidly rising building prices it may be that a particular design cannot be built within these cost limits. If this is likely to be the case then the doctors and their architect should conduct negotiations with the Regional Medical Officer to see whether or not there is some special reason why costs are high (for example a difficult site) and to see whether a special cost limit for the project can be agreed. The need to seek agreement before work is started cannot be over-emphasised.

(iv) Unfortunately, any doctor deciding to build his own purpose-designed premises will find that not only does he need to seek the approval of the health authorities in the guise of the Family Practitioner Committee and Regional Medical Officer, but he also has to satisfy the Local Authority Planning Department. His architect will obviously know how to go about this but occasionally the differing requirements of the two authorities may cause frustration for those not expecting problems.

(v) The doctor, or doctors, involved in the arrangement of the General Practice Finance Corporation loan will need to have some guarantee which they can offer the Corporation over the repayment of their mortgage. Such a guarantee must ensure repayment of the loan should the doctor die prematurely and also provide the capital sum due at the agreed term of the loan. It is usual to negotiate a loan for a period of 20-25 years.

In some cases the doctor undertakes to pay a set interest charge (deducted quarterly by the Family Practitioner Committee, and balanced by the monthly payments of notional rent) throughout the term of the loan. At the end of the term, the capital has to be paid back to the General Practice Finance Corporation. The provision of this capital sum usually requires the individual doctor to arrange some sort of linked life assurance or mortgage protection policy.

In other cases, the doctor undertakes to repay capital and interest (deducted quarterly by the Family Practitioner Committee) so that at the end of the term of the mortgage, the final repayment represents the last part of outstanding loan. With this type of repayment arrangement, there is still a need for insurance, but usually the cheaper mortgage protection type of policy will be sufficient.

Since the sums involved may be quite large, it is important to have skilled advice about the best type of insurance. Endowment assurances with profits may in the long run prove to be the most financially advantageous form, but, for the doctor who may possibly already be financing his own house purchase, the heavy premium payments may mean that some other type of insurance would be more appropriate.

Various insurance companies, including the Medical Sickness Society, have developed special types of policy which combine the traditional endowment assurance with profits with a reducing mortgage protection policy. These companies and most insurance brokers, accountants or bank managers can give advice on such matters, and the General Practice Finance Corporation itself may give helpful ideas to doctors using its service.

(vi) The cost rent scheme was instituted in 1977. A recent amendment has enabled the GPFC to enter into an agreement with a practice to purchase and lease back purpose built, self-contained surgery premises newly completed by the doctors. The scheme is flexible. When considering the capital arrangements needed for new premises practitioners are advised to consider this possibility at an earlier stage. The relevant paragraphs in the Red Book are 51.18.1 to 51.58.23.

(vii) One further charge which the doctors must meet will be the expenses incurred in the day-to-day management of *their* building and the routine maintenance. These items would equate with the service charge made in health centres. Most organised practices will arrange a special account into which a regular sum is paid to underwrite unexpected expenses and redecoration.

(viii) When a doctor joins a practice where there is an existing purpose-built surgery already financed by a loan from the General Practice Finance Corporation there may be problems. These arise usually because the retiring general practitioner or the existing partners require the incoming partner to take a share in the financial responsibility for the freehold property. In this case, the new doctor will be faced both with the possible purchase of his own house and the responsibility of raising a large sum of money to buy into the freehold of the partnership's premises. Most partnerships will try to make this as easy as possible for their new partner but, in spite of this, his initial reaction may be one of fright when he looks at his total borrowing requirements. Nevertheless, he should understand that as far as the practice premises are concerned, he can borrow directly from the General Practice Finance Corporation at their current rate of interest. The conditions of the loan are similar to those described above for doctors building their own premises except that he will have to pay the current rate to the Finance Corporation.

(ix) Paying off the General Practice Finance Corporation and other loans by partnerships is a very complicated affair, especially if the doctors in the partnerships are drawing different percentages of the partnership profits. Some accountants with experience in such matters adjust the capital accounts of each partner annually to balance changes in the assets of the partnership produced by quarterly repayments of capital to the General Practice Finance Corporation.

(c) Premises Rented from Independent Landlords: Special Points of Financing

In the case of premises provided by an independent landlord, if they have been purpose built for the doctors concerned, it is essential that agreement should be reached with the Family Practitioner Committee that the cost rent scheme is applicable before the doctor is committed to renting the premises. The same requirements regarding cost limits will apply if the full rental charge by the landlord is to be refunded as a cost rental from the Family Practitioner Committee. There are some advantages to the system of a private landlord providing premises for a group of doctors. For example, it may be that one or more doctors in a partnership are prepared to finance the premises for the whole partnership, and that the other partners do not wish to be involved in raising money through a mortgage but are prepared to pay a rent for the provision of premises. However, such an arrangement does preclude the non-freeholders from the security provided by property ownership, and from the possibility of a long-term gain in the capital value of the premises in which they work.

2. Improvement of Existing Premises

As the demands made upon a general practice change so the doctors may agree that changes in the existing premises are necessary. Finance to help with improvements may be available either through the cost rent scheme or through an improvement grant. The cost rent scheme is summarised in Section 2 of this chapter. It applies to premises bought and subsequently undergoing substantial modification and to the substantial modification of existing practice premises. Improvement grants are available for the improvement of what exists as opposed to new building or rebuilding. The doctors must have security of tenure. These grants are designed to cover circumstances in which a tax allowance is not available for money spent in alterations. It is essential that practitioners should approach the Family Practitioner Committee before starting work or entering into a contract with a builder for two reasons. Firstly, an improvement grant may or may not be the best way to help finance the operation and the Family Practitioner Committee is in the best position to advise on this. Secondly, that unless prior approval has been obtained from the Family Practitioner Committee no grant will be paid however laudable the project.

The conditions to be fulfilled are contained in paragraphs 56.1 to 56.19 of the Red Book. The Family Practitioner Committee is itself empowered to authorise improvements costing up to £2,650 (1984). Larger applications have also to have approval from the DHSS. The maximum grant per practitioner is £5,300 and there is an overall limit of grant of £18,500 (1984). Paragraph 56, Schedule 2, of the Red Book provides further details.

Further Reading

Department of Health and Social Security. *Health Centres: A Design Guide* (Welsh Office: HMSO, 1970).

Dwyer, D.P.M. 'Converting Practice Premises', chapter in *The Medical Annual, 1983* (Bristol: John Wright).

Scottish Home and Health Department. *Design Guide: Health Centres in Scotland* (London: HMSO, 1973).

Chapter 11: Section 2

Practical Advice on Planning, Building, and Improving Premises

---

STEPS TO BE TAKEN FOR PLANNING/BUILDING NEW PREMISES

STAGE 1

A. *PRACTICE DISCUSSION*

Practice discussion on

- need for new premises
- possible alternatives
- financial implications

Broad planning

- consideration of sites
- consideration of architects

More detailed planning

B. *CONSULT:* • *FPC* for advice re initial acceptability of siting, size and design
• *Local Authority* for advice about planning permission

C. *RECONCILE* VIEWS
DECISION whether to proceed } if Yes → STAGE 2

STAGE 2

D. *SELECTION of site*: initial approach to vendor
of architect: state requirements
agree initial outline

E. *CONSULT: FPC* for approval of preliminary plans
for preliminary estimate of cost rent (with special regard to allowances which may be granted for 'abnormal externals')

F. *NOTIFY* the Regional Medical Officer

G. *APPLY* for outline planning permission from the Local Authority (meetings with Planning Officers)

H. *CAPITAL*: • make preliminary estimate of capital needed
• investigate possible sources of capital
• compare advantages/disadvantages of different methods of repayment
• discuss/agree financial arrangements between partners to include the retirement or death of a partner before repayment has been completed

I. *DECISION* whether to proceed: if YES → STAGE 3

STAGE 3

J. *AGREE with District Valuer* (through FPC) the purchase price of the site which will be allowed for cost rent purposes
with Architect detailed plans
with the FPC the acceptability of the proposed premises for reimbursement under the cost rent scheme; the method for calculating the cost rent to be reimbursed; a preliminary assessment of the cost rent reimbursement: this agreement should be confirmed in a WRITTEN STATEMENT from the FPC

K. *SEND* plans out to tender

L. *DECISION* whether to proceed after consideration of the total cost, the reimbursements agreed, the terms on which the capital can be borrowed and repaid, and the projected running costs of the new building (including insurance): if YES → STAGE 4

STAGE 4

The order in which the actions in this stage are carried out depends on practice circumstances.

M. *CONTRACT* to borrow money
N. *PURCHASE* site
O. *ACCEPT* tender

STAGE 5

During building it is essential for partners to support the architect by keeping a watching brief.

P. *FILE* in order all payments made concerning:
   - land
   - planning and local authority
   - architect
   - builder
   - banks and other financial institutions
   - interest on loans
   - services (e.g. gas, electricity, telephones)

Q. *OBTAIN* completion certificate
R. *MOVE* into completed building: interim cost rent applies from this date
S. *NEGOTIATE* final cost rent with the FPC

STEPS TO BE TAKEN FOR IMPROVEMENT GRANTS

A. *DISCUSSION* in practice on improvements needed and methods of financing
B. *READ* paragraphs 56.1-56.19 of the Red Book
C. *SEEK ADVICE* from the FPC
D. *OBTAIN*:
   - planning permission if needed from landlord or local authority
   - sketch plan of premises and proposed work
   - specification of work to be done
   - estimated total cost

E. *APPLY* to FPC for an improvement grant
F. *RECEIVE* written approval from the FPC before accepting tenders or entering into contracts
G. *ACCEPT* tender/contract

EXAMPLE OF INSTRUCTIONS TO ARCHITECTS

1. That it should not look like an institution (e.g. hospital outpatients health centre) but that the patient should feel comfortable, at home.
2. That the building should require minimal maintenance.
3. That there should be waiting areas/room separated from the entrance and reception area.
4. That one exit from the 'medical' waiting room/area should be directly to a group of consulting rooms.
5. That having seen the doctor the patient should be able to get out of the building by going past the reception desk, but not going through the waiting room/area.
6. That the treatment room and nurses' office should have its own accessible waiting area.
7. That the receptionists 'front area' should have direct communication to the general office containing the records.
8. That incoming telephone calls shall be received so that the replies are not audible in the reception area or to waiting patients.
9. That there shall be a separate secretarial office which is accessible from the general office.
10. That the 'common room' for medical and ancillary staff shall be sited so that combined use is likely. It should have a small adjacent kitchen.
11. That doctors and nurses shall be able to reach the common room/general office without going through the patient waiting area.
12. That separate residential accommodation be provided within the same building (for message-taker).
13. That main rooms and corridors shall all have access to natural light.
14. That the dimensions of the building shall be within the limits accepted by the FPC.
15. That the cost of the building shall be within the accepted current cost limits.
16. That the practice 'domestic' area (office, commonroom, secretaries office, etc.) shall intercommunicate with minimal corridor space.
17. That the building shall be capable of expansion.
18. That the building shall be capable of conversion to private dwellings.
19. That there shall be adequate sound-proofing.

The final design incorporating these instructions is shown in Figure 11.1 overleaf. The first instruction was met by irregular room sizes and corridor widths, arches in the corridors, varying ceiling heights, furnishings, wall lights to supplement overhead lights. Externally a pitched roof and windows of varying size established the buildings' non-institutional character.

Figure 11.1: Final Architect's Design for New Premises

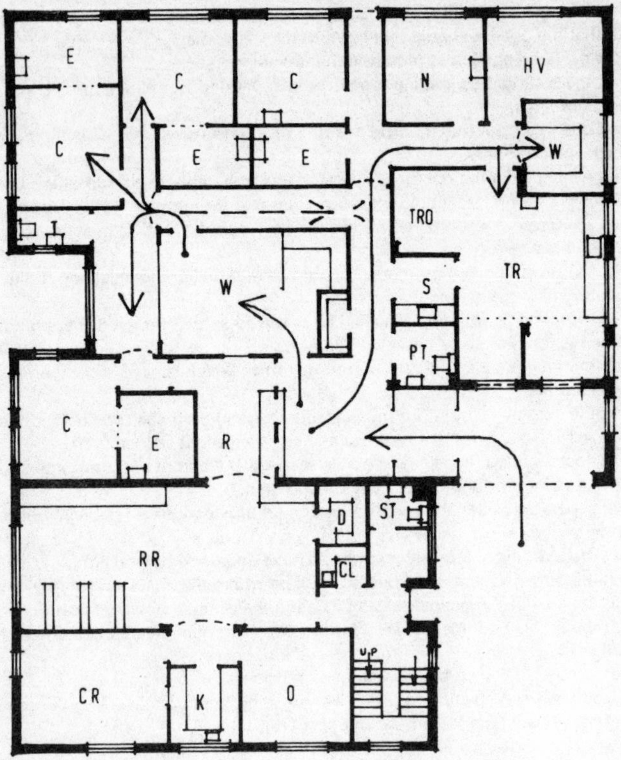

KEY:—

- - -	ARCH
C	CONSULTING ROOM
CL	CLEANER
CR	COMMON ROOM
D	DRUG STORE
E	EXAMINATION ROOM
HV	HEALTH VISITOR
K	KITCHEN
N	NURSES ROOM
O	OFFICE
PT	PATIENTS' TOILET
R	RECEPTION OFFICE
RR	RECORDS/RECEPTION AREA
S	SLUICE ROOM
ST	STAFF TOILET
T	TOILET
TR	TREATMENT ROOM
TRO	TREATMENT OFFICE
W	WAITING AREA

PART FOUR:

PAPERS

12 CONTRACTS

Introduction

Becoming a principal in general practice involves undertaking formal relationships with many different organisations and people. They include:

(a) A contract with the Family Practitioner Committee.
(b) A contract with individual patients.
(c) A contract with partners.
(d) A contract with each employee.
(e) Contracts with landlords (or, for those working in owner-occupied premises, mortgages and/or loan agreements).
(f) Contracts with insurance companies.

(a) The Contract with the Family Practitioner Committee

Many doctors find it difficult to understand what is meant by 'independent contractor'. In fact, it is the common state for most senior professionals, and only since the National Health Service led to the introduction of salaried consultants in 1948 was the situation altered. Until that time most doctors, lawyers and accountants were self-employed independent contractors offering their services in return for a fee. For general practitioners, that situation continues except that the Secretary of State for Health and Social Security has underwritten the patient's obligation to pay a fee. The significance and consequences of the independent-contractor status for general practice and general practitioners have been further discussed in Chapter 2.

When he signs his contract with a Family Practitioner Committee on becoming a principal, the general practitioner states the area in which he is to practise, the premises from which he intends to practise, the hours available for consultation, and the name and address of any other doctor with whom he intends to practise. He agrees to provide certain services (general medical, maternity, contraceptive). The regulations lay down that these shall be 'necessary and appropriate personal medical services of the type usually provided by general practitioners'. In return for providing these services he is entitled to National Health Service fees and allowances.

(b) The Contract with the Patient

Each person is issued with a National Health Service medical card (FP.4). This card forms the basis of a tripartite contract; a contract between the patient and the doctor in which the doctor agrees to provide services, and a contract between the doctor and the Family Practitioner Committee acting as the agent of the District Health Authority in which the latter contracts to pay the doctor the current fees as laid down in the Red Book. On his part, the doctor contracts with the Family Practitioner Committee that he will fulfil the terms and conditions of service regarding the provision of medical services as far as that particular patient is concerned. The contract between the doctor and the patient is therefore a personal one, just as the relationship between the doctor and his patient is also personal.

Most patients who join a doctor's list present the doctor with their medical cards. Some will not be able to find their medical cards. These patients should be given a form (FP.1) which they complete and present in place of a medical card. When patients register the birth of newly born infants they are given a small pink card (FP.58) by the Registrar of Births and Deaths which fulfils the same purpose as a medical card. This is given to the doctor when he accepts the infant on his list.

When patients present the doctor or his receptionist with their medical card it is important to check that they have completed and signed either Parts A or B of the card. When a new patient registers many practices use the opportunity to provide a practice information leaflet giving details of surgery times and special clinics together with other general information about the practice to the new patients. Some doctors like to see all their new patients, partly to emphasise the personal nature of the doctor/patient relationship, but often also to record basic background information on a medical record card.

Once the medical card has been received by the doctor or his receptionist, the doctor must sign the card and date it. This signifies his acceptance of the patient on his list. He should also enter whether or not he is to supply drugs to the patient. If he is entitled to claim rural practice payments then he should enter the mileage in the space provided. The completed card is then sent to the Family Practitioner Committee.

(c) The Contract with Partners

There is nothing quite like a happy partnership. Doctors in such a group know that they do not need formal agreements to keep them happy; but sensible general practitioners know that when things go wrong a properly drawn partnership deed can save distress and embarrassment to everyone.

No one should enter into partnership anticipating trouble. Ideally, a partnership should be a progressive association of colleagues and friends, but agreed rules at the start may help determine how the relationships develop and can determine what happens if they break down. It is much easier to draw up the governing rules of the partnership before rather than after the partnership begins. It is better still to have them written in legal form from the start. However, solicitors work at their own speed and often formal deeds cannot be prepared in time to meet the start of the partnership. If the rules are agreed, an exchange of letters of intent between the doctors involved and their solicitors is usually a satisfactory guarantee, provided the letters also include a date by which the partnership documents must be signed.

Which Solicitor?

Most solicitors are prepared to draw up partnership agreements but some are much more experienced in this work than others. Frequently, medical groups will ask solicitors used to preparing medical partnership deeds to act for them. The Personal Services Bureau of the BMA issues an advisory leaflet on partnership agreements (Medical Partnerships under the National Health Service) and is willing to inspect members' draft agreeements and advise on them.

How Much Does it Cost?

A properly drawn partnership agreement is not a cheap document, and may cost several hundred pounds. In the event of later disagreement it can save many thousands of pounds.

What is Covered?

The agreement should cover every aspect of doctors working together, the rules governing both the day-to-day working of the practice and long-term practice policy. It should specify the arrangements for the medical policy and management of the practice as well as the appointment of staff.

It should set out how the rota for on-call, holidays, sick leave and study leave is drawn up, and must lay down rules covering the financial arrangement for the practice — not only where money earned comes from (and what exactly is partnership money) but how and when shares are paid to individual doctors. Financial clauses should cover such things as tax liability, ownership of partnership property (both freehold and leasehold), liability for rented accommodation, and the capital assets of the firm.

The arrangements for retirement must be agreed, and the procedure to be followed in case of the death or chronic illness of a partner stated. It is essential to set out how and for what reasons the partnership may be dissolved. The more comprehensive the partnership deed the more it is likely to cost *but* in the event of disagreement between partners, the easier the solution.

The following is a check list covering items which appear in most partnership deeds:

(1) *Who?* Who are to form the medical partnership? What is its name?

(2) *When?* When does it start, how long may it continue? Does anyone have a fixed date or age of retirement?

(3) *Where?* Where does the medical partnership practise, is there a defined area?

(4) *What?* What notice must a partner give if he wishes to leave?

(5) *Holidays.* How many days (or weeks) are allowed each year? Who has first choice (or is it by rota?)

(6) *Study and Sabbatical Leave.* These need to be specified.

(7) *Sick Leave.* Sick leave rights need to be stated since ill health of one partner throws both an increased workload and an increased financial burden on the remaining partners. Must partners have an agreed minimum sickness insurance? Who pays for it, the partnership or the individual doctor? Who gets it? Who pays

for a locum if needed? What is the partnership policy with regard to money received under the National Health Service sickness benefit scheme? How long will the partnership allow a sick member to continue as a partner?

(8) *Money In.* It is essential to specify precisely what constitutes 'partnership money' and what is the individual doctor's own money. For example, does every professional fee go to the partnership (what about lecture fees earned on a partner's half-day or weekend off or money earned during holidays)? How is the scale of private fees of the partnership determined? What is a *Gift* and what is a 'payment for professional service'? What about legacies, are these ever equivalent to professional receipts? Seniority and vocational training payments are individually earned by a doctor, but are they to go into the partnership pool or not? If they are, who is to benefit from the superannuation which goes with them, the individual who earned them or everyone?

(9) *Money Out.* Which bank holds the partnership accounts and who signs the cheques? What expenses are to be met by the partnership and how is the remainder to be divided? Is there to be immediate parity for a new partner, or is this to be gradually attained? What about car expenses and telephone expenses?

(10) *Accountancy.* How is income and expenditure to be recorded, what are the accounting days and who is to prepare the partnership accounts?

(11) *On Duty and Off Duty.* How is the partnership's National Health Service practice preserved (e.g. no partner may withdraw from night or weekend duty, and no partner may do anything to prejudice his receipt of a basic practice allowance)? Are equal shares to be paid for equal work? Do senior (or older) partners drop money when they drop duty?

(12) *Precedence.* Do senior partners have privileges and, if so, what are they and are these reasonable?

(13) *Partnership Meetings.* Are these to be held regularly? How is the chairman appointed, and does the post rotate amongst all partners? Are minutes to be kept?

(14) *Administration.* What management jobs are to be allocated to partners (e.g. finance, staffing, building and maintenance) and do they rotate?

(15) *Miscellaneous.*

(a) Where may partners live?

(b) If a partner moves, who pays increased telephone

costs? (e.g. for an extended direct line from the practice switchboard).

(c) If a partner leaves, must he covenant not to set up in opposition practice within a defined area? How much does he pay if he breaks this covenant?

(d) Is there an agreed selection procedure for new partners?

(e) Should there be a clause covering arbitration where partners fail to agree, e.g. over the valuation of freehold property when a retiring partner is leaving?

(f) Representative appointments (service on the LMC etc.) are often looked upon as a responsibility (and honour) for the practice. Is the serving partner to be covered during his absence by the remaining partners?

(g) Outside appointments are quite common. What is the practice policy in respect of new appointments? Does the agreement need to refer to this? Can a partner give up an existing appointment without the consent of his partners (practice income may fall)?

(h) Is it necessary to have a special rule to cover the possibility of a partner being called up for National Service in Her Majesty's Armed Forces?

(i) Is membership of the Medical Defence Union or Medical Protection Society or a similar organisation obligatory?

(j) Are partners allowed to engage in other businesses (e.g. can one become a farmer)?

(k) Does the agreement specifically state that personal debts may not be secured against partnership assets (without the written consent of all the partners)?

(16) It is usual for the deed to state that 'all shall employ themselves diligently in the practice and use their utmost endeavours' and go on to state that 'each shall be faithful and just one to the other'. Finally, all agree to share the cost of the preparation of the deed.

With the current difficulty in obtaining principal posts, and with an increasing number of unpleasant consequences of partnership breakdowns being reported to the GMC, considerable interest has recently been taken in the matter of partnership agreements. A general review may be found in the third edition of *The Business of General Practice 1983/84* published by Medical Publications Ltd and distributed by the GMSC. Problems which are commonly encountered within partnerships are considered and possible solutions discussed in Appendix 11 of the General Medical Services Committee's Report to the Annual Conference of Representatives of Local Medical Committees 1984.

Clearly, legal documents — however comprehensive and however pious the clauses — cannot make a medical partnership work. It is the spirit with which each doctor enters into partnership which ensures success or failure.

(d) The Contract with Staff

In some practices each doctor has an individual secretary/receptionist who gets to know the working habits, outside commitments and rate of consultation of her particular doctor. This makes for a good working relationship but has the disadvantage of producing problems during holidays, sickness and other leave. It also presumes that the secretary is going to be available all day for that particular doctor. A more efficient system for the average practice is to try and make all reception staff virtually interchangeable so that they can all receive patients, take telephone calls and file records at various times. If this system is used then there should still be one member of staff who does most of the secretarial work with another member of staff to back her up in the case of her absence. For each employee a job description should be part of her contract.

The terms of service of staff will depend on the needs of the practice, but for part-time staff, hourly rates of pay are usual. These should be reviewed annually and incremental increases in line with nationally accepted norms considered. Guidance for rates of pay for secretaries and nurses can be obtained by reference to comparable hospital or health authority rates. Sick leave and holiday arrangements vary from practice to practice, but it is usual for most staff to have three to four weeks' paid holiday.

It is a good principle to pay good staff well. Reception staff who are well trained and can deal correctly with patients should be highly valued. Their cost to the doctors is small when weighed against the beneficial effect they have on the practice. Moreover the 30 per cent of their salaries which is not reimbursed is tax deductible.

When appointing new staff it should be made quite clear to them what their hours will be, any holiday relief work expected, their rate of pay, number of weeks' holiday and sick-leave allowance. Above all the importance of confidentiality of information should be emphasised. A gossiping receptionist can soon damage the practice's reputation.

For further training of staff, the Association of Medical Secretaries may be helpful. This organisation holds local meetings and annual symposia. Doctors may consider taking their staff with them to medical meetings in practice organisation, and for reading material an introductory book is *The Medical Secretary's Handbook* by Michael Drury (1981).

Contracts of Employment for Staff

Since the Employment Protection Act of 1975 each employer has had specific obligations to his employees. This Act affects every practitioner, even if he only employs one person. The rights and obligations involved are as follows:

1. Particulars of Employment. The Act lays down that particulars of the contract of employment must be given in writing to all employees with three exceptions:

(a) Where the employee is the husband or wife.

(b) Where an employee engaged since 1 January 1976 is employed for less than 16 hours per week.

(c) Where an employee who had by then worked for five years continuously is employed for less than eight hours per week.

The particulars, which can be given by letter or in any other written form, must include (a) salary, (b) job title, (c) holiday entitlement, (d) sick leave and pay, (e) period of notice, (f) right to redundancy payment, (g) rights against unfair dismissal, (h) right of union membership, (i) disciplinary rules and (j) grievance procedure.

2. Itemised Pay Statement. The employer must itemise his employee's pay statement so that it shows gross wages or salary, deductions (and for what purposes they are made) and the net pay.

3. Notice. After four weeks of continuous employment, an employee can be dismissed only by notice so that a practitioner must decide in that initial period whether to dismiss an employee summarily.

Between the four weeks' qualifying period and 24 months of continuous employment, one weeks' notice of termination of employment must be given. After two years, the employee is entitled to one week's notice for each completed year of employment up to a maximum of twelve weeks.

Notice should always be given in writing.

4. Dismissal. Every person who has been employed for a minimum of 26 weeks has a right not to be unfairly dismissed, subject to there being a minimum number of employees in the business (currently four). If an employee is unsatisfactory, he or she must be given a proper warning and an opportunity to improve. If things are still unsatisfactory, a final warning in writing must be given. If there seems to be no alternative to dismissal, the employee must be given a proper opportunity to state his or her case and can then be given written notice of termination. The employee can call upon the employer to give a written statement of reasons for dismissal though, in practice, it is advisable to incorporate the reasons in the notice of dismissal.

An aggrieved employee can apply to an Industrial Tribunal for compensation to be paid by the employer. Resignation as an alternative to dismissal counts as dismissal and enables a disgruntled employee to take proceedings.

5. Maternity. Associated with the general right against unfair dismissal are a female employee's additional rights:

(a) Not to be dismissed because of pregnancy without being first offered suitable alternative employment.

(b) To be given six weeks' maternity pay provided she works until eleven weeks before her estimated date of confinement and has at that time completed two years' continuous service.

(c) To return to her job within 29 weeks of confinement.

6. Redundancy. A person who has been employed for a minimum of 104 weeks and who is dismissed because of cessation of business (such as closure of a practice) is entitled to a redundancy payment calculated according to a statutory formula. The employer can claim rebate of one half of the sum paid from the State Redundancy Payment Fund, and the balance (or a proportion of the balance if the member of staff is employed only partly on qualifying duties) from the Family Practitioner Committee.

7. Liability for Accidents at Work. All employers are liable for accidents to employees caused by defective equipment, leaving the employer in appropriate cases to claim an indemnity from the manufacturer. Employers must also insure against claims by employees for accidents occurring to them in the course of their work.

8. Sex Discrimination. An employer must not discriminate against a married or unmarried person of either sex in the arrangements he makes for determining who will be offered employment. There are separate provisions relating to advertising. A practitioner must distinguish between applicants for a job by their ability only and should in advertising make it clear that a post is open to members of either sex.

9. Equal pay. Men and women in the same employment must be treated equally in terms of pay so long as the woman's and the man's work are of the same nature in terms of effort, skill and decision. This applies, for instance, to a practice employing two part-time managers, one a man and one a woman, in that if their duties are comparable they must be paid equally.

10. Union Membership. An employee is entitled to belong to a Trade Union and to take part in its activities outside working hours without interference from the employer.

Statutory Sick Pay

The social Security and Housing Benefits Act (1982) introduced many changes in sickness benefit. Practitioners will all be aware of the changes in certification rules which affect them as providers of certificates. They may not be aware of their obligations as employers, and the fact that since 6 April 1983 they have been responsible for paying Statutory Sick Pay to those employees who fall sick for a maximum period of eight weeks in any tax year. The procedures are complex. Fines for not observing the regulations range from £200 to £1,000 or a term of imprisonment.

Practitioners are strongly advised to obtain some sickness records sheets (SSP2), other relevant forms (SSP1(T) and SSP1(E)) and the *Employers Guide to Statutory Sick Pay* from their local DHSS office. They are also strongly advised to ensure that someone within the practice, such as the senior secretary or practice manager, understands the practice's obligations and is responsible for seeing they are carried out. A flow chart and diagram which show the outline of the scheme can be found in Section 2 of this chapter.

(e) Contract with Landlords or Mortgagor

Most doctors will either rent their practice accommodation (and have a contract with a landlord) or own their premises.

In the case of doctors in rented premises, the landlord may either be the District Health Authority or an independent private landlord.

The Model Health Centre licence (sent by the Department of Health and Social Security to all Area Health Authorities in April 1977) forms a basis on which doctors who practise from health centres may make a contract with the District Health Authority.

Contracts with private landlords are individually arranged. Good legal advice is essential when drawing up such a contract.

General practitioners who work from their own premises usually have a mortgage or a loan from either the General Practice Finance Corporation or from a Building Society. In either case, a further contract is inevitable. A fuller description of the methods of financing premises and the agreements required is given in Chapter 11.

(f) Contracts Covering Insurance

Apart from life insurance and mortgage protection, general practitioners as independent contractors need to insure themselves against claims from staff or patients who may be injured on the practice premises. These are termed Employer's Liability and Public Liability insurance. In addition, a doctor's full insurance against medical malpractice is essential and should be a condition of joining a partnership.

General practitioners have full-time responsibility for patient care. They have particular need for insurance against absence through sickness, especially since the sickness of a partner may entail the employment of a locum practitioner. Some companies are prepared to give permanent sickness cover specially adapted to the needs of doctors in partnership. It is usual for partners to insure also against consequential loss through general insurances covering the practice premises and contents.

Insurance is such an important subject that most general practitioners will need specialist advice. The services of an insurance broker used to dealing with the needs of family doctors may be useful, or advice from the Medical Insurance Agency or the Medical Sickness Annuity and Life Assurance Society Limited should be sought.

Breaking Contracts

No one really enters into a contract with the object of breaking it. However, for all sorts of reasons it is sometimes necessary to terminate contracts. All legal agreements should have a clause which clearly sets out the procedure to be followed if the contract is to be terminated. It is as well to be aware of the rules when entering into a contract.

If the delicate relationship between doctor and patient is broken, the contract which the doctor entered into with the Family Practitioner Committee and the patient will have to be ended. There is a set procedure for doing this.

The doctor may notify the FPC that he wishes a certain patient to be removed from his list and, provided the patient is not under medical treatment at the time, the patient is removed from the practitioner's list after seven days. The doctor does not have to give reasons for his request.

The patient has similar rights. He may inform the FPC that he wishes to be removed from the doctor's list (or change to another doctor). With the written consent of his doctor he may change immediately to another practitioner, provided the second practitioner agrees, otherwise he must give fourteen days' notice of his decision to be removed from his doctor's list.

We believe that the doctor has a duty to his patient to consider whether or not the breakdown in relationships is a symptom of the patient's ill-health and, if so, whether or not steps to heal the breach would be more in keeping with the proper role of the practitioner. Only in the very last resort should doctors remove patients from their list. It is an admission of failure but it happens occasionally to all of us.

Disciplinary Procedure

Occasionally, following a breakdown in relations between a doctor and his patient, a complaint is made. This complaint is made to the Family Practitioner Committee by the patient. It may be formal or informal.

In the case of formal complaints there is a medical service procedure which has to be followed. All principals in general practice should be aware of the complaints procedure which patients may use against them. No one enters practice contemplating being subject to disciplinary procedure, but it can happen unexpectedly.

The commonest cause of complaint is 'failure to visit' and doctors who have been subject to this complaint often wonder why it happened; usually the reason is a failure in communication between doctor and patient. The doctor who may have said on the telephone, 'I think the problem is so and so and if you do such and such, the situation will improve' — may have meant to add, 'If it doesn't, let me know and I'll come,' but this has been construed by the patient as 'doctor refused to come'. Hence the complaint.

The Administrator (or his deputy) and the Chairman of the Family Practitioner Committee will usually try and sort out most complaints informally. They will try to find out what each side thinks happened and then try to settle the matter amicably between the parties concerned. If the complaint is apparently serious, or the complaining patient or doctor demands a formal hearing, then the Administrator of the Family Practitioner Committee must arrange for a hearing before the Medical Services Committee.

The procedure of a medical services committee is complicated. For detailed advice and information the doctor is advised to contact his medical defence organisation. Both the Medical Defence Union and the Medical Protection Society publish advisory booklets which members receive on request.

Further Reading

Complaints to Family Practitioner Committees (Medical Defence Union, London, 1975).
Employing Staff Ellis, Norman (London: BMA Publications, 1984).
Law and the Doctor (Medical Defence Union, London, 1977).
Medical Partnerships under the National Health Service (BMA Personal Services Bureau, 1976).
Pitfalls and Worries of the Young Doctor (Medical Protection Society, London).
Professional Conduct and Discipline (General Medical Council, London, 1977).

Chapter 12: Section 2

A. Example of a Contract with Staff from a Three-partner Practice

---

CONTRACT OF EMPLOYMENT
Agreement between
Drs. AND ....

Date of Commencement of Employment:
Title of Job:

Working Hours:	Your appointment with the Practice is on a monthly basis and your hours of work are: Monday Tuesday Wednesday Thursday Friday Saturday. You may be expected to work additional or different hours during staff holidays, but any alteration of hours due to sickness of any other member of staff will be with your agreement.
Holiday Entitlement:	You will be entitled to 4 weeks holiday (January to January) with pay. All holidays must be agreed with the Employer not less than two weeks in advance and all holidays must be taken during the year in respect of which they are due. Holidays should not coincide with those of other employees of the Practice. In the event of such coincidence the person with the longest term of continuous employment shall have first choice of dates. Any period of holiday taken should be for at least one week.
Salary:	Your salary will be paid in arrears monthly by cheque. There are no Pension rights attached to this employment and there is no contracting out certificate in force under the Social Security Pensions Act 1975. Increments are paid in of each year.
Salary:	After one year's employment absence due to sickness will be on a full pay less the usual deductions for three weeks and thereafter at the discretion of the Practice. You are expected to produce a Medical Certificate to cover periods of sickness.

Grievance Procedure:	You should raise any grievance relating to your employment with any of the Partners, however Dr X must be informed. Minor grievances may be raised orally but serious grievances must be expressed in writing.
Termination of Employment:	One month's written notice of termination of employment is required by both employee and employer except that break of confidentiality or gross misconduct will result in instant dismissal.
Retirement:	Retirement age for Women is 60 though an extension may be arranged by mutual agreement.
Accidents:	Any accident occurring on the premises to staff or a visitor must be reported to a partner as soon as possible.
Disciplinary Rules:	You accept that all information you see or hear is confidential and must not be disclosed to unauthorised persons. Failure to observe this will constitute grounds for summary dismissal.

I accept this appointment on the terms and conditions mentioned above.

Signed .... *EMPLOYEE*

DATE ....SIGNED .... *EMPLOYER*

N.B. The British Medical Association has produced a model staff contract which is available to members. Practitioners are strongly advised to study this as a basis for contracts with their staff.

B. Statutory Sick Pay Procedure

Figure 12.1 (overleaf) summarises the steps an employer should take when an employee is sick.

Figure 12.1: Procedure for Statutory Sick Pay

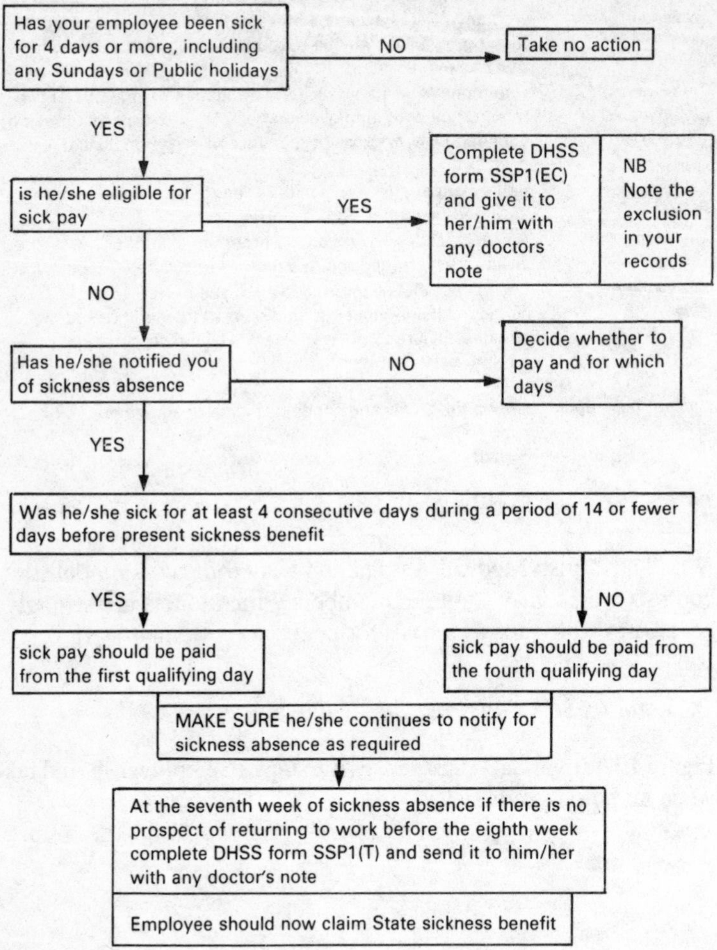

N.B. As an employer you are *obliged by law* to keep records of sick pay paid to individuals and the total amount paid in each tax year *you should therefore keep records of*

1. All periods of 'incapacity for work' for periods of more than four days (whether the employee would have worked on those days, e.g. Sunday, or not).
2. Any day recorded in the period of incapacity for which statutory sick pay (SSP) was not paid.
3. Reasons for not paying the sick pay.
4. Details of each employee's 'qualifying days' in each period of sickness within the tax year.

(A 'qualifying day', to be agreed between employer and employee is a day on which an employee normally works.)

13 RECORDS

Record-keeping has always been one of the weaker aspects of general practice. Even now many general practitioners maintain that they can practise good medicine without writing in the patient's notes, relying on their memory and relationship with the patient. It is only over the past twenty years, with the example set by doctors such as Keith Hodgkin and John Fry, that interest has been stimulated in this field so that some new form of record-keeping seems to be reported every few months. In 1972 Dawes surveyed eight practices and considered the data recorded to be of poor quality. In 50 per cent of episodes no diagnosis was entered, in 10 per cent a diagnosis was recorded without supporting evidence. Less than half contained information about symptoms. Physical signs were only mentioned in one third of cases.

There are many reasons for keeping a record from merely using it as an *aide-mémoire* to major practice research activities. Whatever the reason in an individual practice there is no doubt that doctors offering primary care in the 1980s cannot claim to have an efficient record system if it is not capable of:

- (i) Identifying patients by age and sex.
- (ii) Indicating the last attendance for a patient and the reason for this together with the action taken.
- (iii) Showing the relevant features of patient's past medical history.
- (iv) Indicating the patient's weight, blood pressure, smoking and drinking habits.
- (v) Indicating relevant immunisation and vaccination history and other aspects of preventive care such as cervical smears.
- (vi) Identifying major disease groups with a list of the patients in the practice suffering from those conditions.
- (vii) Recalling identified groups of patients for routine preventive care activities such as developmental assessment, cervical smears or blood pressure check.
- (viii) A built-in audit system to monitor workload and patient care.

This is not an impractical list as many general practitioners in the country already have systems capable of meeting most or all of these requirements. Records will be considered in three groups.

1. The patient record
2. Registers
3. Recall Systems

Only manual systems using written records will be considered as computers are dealt with in Chapter 14.

1. The Patient Record

Three main types of record are found in general practice:

(a) Medical Record Envelope (FP5 and 6)

This envelope has had little modification since it was introduced in 1911. It is the property of the DHSS and is returned to the Family Practitioner Committee after the patient's death. Its small size (7¼ in. × 5 in.) is a major disadvantage. Writing tends to be cramped and illegible, but, even more important, hospital letters and other records rarely fit the envelope without being folded several times. The envelope rapidly becomes bulky, and there is a tendency for doctors not to refer to documents which have been unfolded and refolded.

(b) A4 Folder

This record is based on paper of A4 size (11¾ × 8¼ in.). First introduced in two practices in Wantage (Hawkey *et al.*, 1971; Loudon, 1975), a record folder was designed which has a pocket on the inside of the front of the folder, and a second pocket on the back. Record sheets of A4 size are attached by tags or soft metal strip to two spines which run along the back of the folder. One major advantage of using a folder of A4 size is that hospital reports and correspondence can be filed flat. A second advantage is that the practitioner has more scope and space to organise the record.

An A4 record, however, takes up one and a half times the space of the present envelope. Curtis in 1974 surveyed 130 general practitioners and found that 48 per cent would not have sufficient space to store A4 records.

So, although in 1973 the DHSS agreed in principle to the conversion of general practice records to A4 (ECN 946 1973), little progress has been made in view of the potential cost of the structural changes which would be needed to store them. The secretarial cost of transferring the traditional record to A4 has been calculated as occupying one secretary up to two years to transfer the records of one principal. Finally, the problem of adapting an A4 record to one of the traditional size when a patient moves from one practice to another has been encountered. The introduction of A4 records has understandably been slow.

(c) Family Folder

Another system is that in which all records of one family are stored together. They are made available whenever one member presents himself or herself. This has some advantages in practices where patients frequently see different doctors, but is probably not justified in other practices as family record may rapidly become very bulky.

Order out of Chaos

In many practices, even in training practices, the patient record is chaotic. When a patient is seen by a doctor other than his own (partners, locums, trainees) the 'record' may consist of well-nigh illegible jottings with sheets and hospital letters all jumbled up together. To enter information in a problem-orientated way is one method of structuring the records so that salient facts are more easily found. But there are other simpler methods of bringing order out of chaos, some of which can be carried out by the office staff, others which need the doctor's attention.

(i) Notes Arranged in Chronological Order. It is relatively simple to arrange the record cards in order. Stapling and sellotape, popular in the past, have in many practices given way to punching a hole and using Treasury tags. With this method inserts or summary cards can be added with little effort. One of the advantages of carrying out this exercise is that the point where the previous record ended will be obvious to anyone making a fresh note, which helps to eliminate all the partly filled EC7s which fatten most record envelopes.

(ii) Letters and Reports Arranged in Order. Again it is a fairly

simple task to arrange these in chronological order. Problems arise with selection. Some doctors hoard every scrap of information in case some test or nuance in a letter which is not relevant at the time might be relevant later. Others are more brutal and abstract without misgiving. If this task is delegated to office staff it is important that the views of each individual doctor are known and respected for the records of his patients.

(iii) Colour Codes on Record Envelopes. The Royal College of General Practitioners has agreed a colour code for certain diseases. Patients with significant conditions can be readily identified by a colour tag on their envelopes to alert the doctor when they are seen.

The same system of record tagging can be used for any other condition or situation which the doctor may wish to identify. The RCGP study on an Attitudes to Pregnancy Survey, for example, requires a tag with APS to be fixed to the outside of the record envelope. In large practices dealing with 15,000-30,000 patients it may be administratively easier to identify each doctor's patients by giving each doctor a colour code and the displayed edge of the record carries this colour. Alternatively each alphabetical shelf may have a different colour so that misplaced records can be easily identified.

(iv) Emphasising Important Facts. Much of the written record is of a descriptive or provisional nature. There are, however, in all records certain diagnoses or procedures which are potentially relevant to any future consultation as an *aide-mémoire* or classifier. Colour coding the envelope has limited possibilities. If important facts are underlined, boxed, or starred on the record itself, then they are less likely to be overlooked.

(v) Summary Cards. A logical extension of boxing or underlining important facts on the record is for these facts to be gathered together on a summary card. Priority details might include diagnoses, operations and drug sensitivities. Summary cards which the doctor can adapt for his own use can be obtained from the Family Practitioner Service. Maycock and colleagues (1979) have described a comprehensive system based on overprinting. Tait, (1977) has described a system using specially printed cards. Summary cards can also be obtained from the Royal College of

General Practitioners.

When the records are in order and summary cards completed it is vital that these systems are then kept updated either by the doctor or by reception staff with the task specifically delegated to them. It is no good making a major push to get the records in order and summarised if over the next few years they become disorganised or outdated. Constant vigilance has to be maintained.

Some doctors are particularly enthusiastic about structuring their records in a problem orientated fashion (POMR). While the complete POMR requires a certain amount of dedication on the part of all doctors and staff, nevertheless there are aspects of it which are vulnerable to all. In order that the reader may decide what is most appropriate for him or her, the full POMR system is described.

Problem Orientated Medical Record (POMR)

This type of record is known as 'problem orientated' because the whole record is based on the problems which patients have. It was originally introduced by Lawrence Weed in 1969 in the USA for hospital records. There are three basic components.

(a) The problem list
(b) Background information package
(c) Plan and progress notes

(a) The Problem List. When a patient first attends, his problems are identified and numbered, for example:

1. Acute bronchitis
2. Rheumatoid arthritis
3. Poor housing

All information in a POMR is entered, stored, retrieved, and used according to the problem to which it refers. When a problem has been resolved this is indicated on the problem list and ceases to be an active problem. For example, P3 — rehoused — satisfactory.

The doctor only needs to deal with the problems presented to him on any one occasion by the patient. If there is no new information on other problems these are left unchanged. The advantage of a problem list organised in this way is that the system reminds the doctor of the unresolved problems at each consultation.

(b) The Background Information Package. This information again is usually obtained when the patient joins the practice list, although some doctors advise collecting it gradually. It has two components, the fixed and the changing information.

(i) The Fixed Information — this consists of:
Sex
Date of birth
Previous illnesses
Immunisation
Family history if relevant

(ii) The Changing Information — this consists of:
Marital status
Occupation
Address
Screening tests, e.g. cervical smear

This package is recorded separately and will obviously not need to be referred to on all occasions.

Some confusion arises between the phrases 'background information package' and 'data base'. The phrase 'data base' was originally used by Weed in its hospital context to include all the information in the 'background information package' plus the results of clinical examinations and laboratory tests.

(c) The Plan & Progress Notes: SOAP. The progress notes are written for each current episode of attendance and only differ from normal record entries in being structured. The patient's complaint is dealt with under the headings:

(i) Subjective — the patient's observations and complaints
(ii) Objective — the results of examinations and investigations
(iii) Analysis — a concise statement of the situation as the doctor sees it
(iv) Plan — this consists of four components:

A. The goal or aim: to try and write down a realistic possible achievement, i.e. to get the diastolic BP below 100 in six weeks.

B. Information required, e.g. the health visitor to check on accommodation.
C. Action — whether and what prescription was given, certificates, etc.
D. Patient education — note, verbatim if possible, what the patient has been told about his condition.

The advantages of writing the current entry in this way are that the doctor is obliged to structure his activities and actions logically. If another doctor sees the patient it is immediately apparent what plans the previous doctor had for action.

Secondary Uses for POMR

1. Quality control of patient care. There is a record of the doctor's thoughts and decisions. Later these can be compared against outcome by the doctor himself to modify his future action.
2. Education. If a medical student or trainee records in the SOAP pattern it is much easier to follow the logic (or absence of logic) of his actions. It is therefore a valuable teaching tool.
3. Preventive medicine. The construction of the background information package enables one to see risk factors for the patient, such as incomplete immunisation schedules.
4. Research. For a researcher doing a retrospective study of records the information is structured and readily identifiable.

2. Registers

The Age/Sex Register

No practice can offer organised preventive care to its population without an age/sex register. This records all the patients in the practice by their year of birth and their sex. It immediately gives the opportunity to list groups such as the under fives (for developmental assessment), the over seventy-fives (at risk group), or ten-year-old girls (for their rubella injection).

The record can be established by either using a loose-leaf folder with one page or more per year and entering the names of patients on the sheet or by using a card index system such as that provided by the Royal College of General Practitioners.

The advantage of the card system is that each card represents a patient and can be tagged and used in a variety of ways besides just for the age/sex information.

Disease Register

It is no good general practitioners claiming that they can offer adequate care to special disease groups such as asthmatics, diabetics or hypertensives if these patients cannot be identified within the practice and their care monitored.

An extensive disease register is probably beyond the scope of most practices but limited and valuable information may be obtained from colour tagging the edge of the age/sex cards so that patients suffering from specific conditions may be identified by looking down the register. There is an agreed universal coding for diseases which is:

Red	— Sensitivity reaction	Black	— Suicide attempt
Yellow	— Epilepsy	Green	— TB
Brown	— Diabetes	Mauve	— Cancer
Blue	— Hypertension		

Practices who wish to be more ambitious can develop a register which was called an E book when first described. Full details of this and other registers can be found in Eimerl & Laidlaw (1969).

3. Recall Systems

Preventive care has been mentioned a number of times and, of course, this is one of the major values of having record systems of the type already described.

Without a computer the number of recall systems which the practice can offer is limited but certainly should include ones for cervical smears, FP1001/1002 (contraceptive record), immunisations and child care. Simple card index systems can be used in conjunction with the age/sex register which will, for instance, give the names of all the girls of 10 due rubella vaccinations, or women over 35 due to have a smear.

Repeat Prescribing

Repeat prescribing is a 'way of life' for the British general practitioner and not commonly found in other health care systems. The reasons for this are varied and complex.

Doctors are under constant pressure from the DHSS to keep their prescribing costs down, and one of the main areas of contention is repeat prescribing with claims that many prescriptions are issued repeatedly without due regard for their necessity. The pharmacists who have to dispense the prescriptions claim that a very high proportion are completed by ancillary staff rather than doctors and that many are inaccurate or incomplete.

Balint was the first to draw attention to other more subtle reasons for issuing repeat prescriptions and identified the patient who needs to have contact with the doctor through a prescription request but is often reluctant to actually consult him. If this delicate relationship is disturbed by the refusal of a repeat prescription or an attempt to change it then a disturbed pattern of doctor/patient relationship develops for a period before settling down into a new repeat prescription pattern.

Whatever the many and varied reasons for repeat prescribing in British general practice, there is no doubt that the doctors concerned do have a professional responsibility to see that their system is efficient, reliable, and not abused.

The groups of drugs prescribed by repeat prescription can be divided as follows:

(i) Those necessary for routine maintenance of chronic conditions. This is the group for which there is little disagreement about issuing some repeat prescriptions and includes treatment for illnesses like hypertension, diabetes or osteoarthritis.

(ii) Those necessary for occasional use. This group includes prescriptions for conditions such as hay fever or migraine which again can be justified provided that the original diagnosis was confirmed by the general practitioner.

(iii) Those originally prescribed by the general practitioner and their continuing use determined by the patient. This is probably the group which causes most debate when discussing repeat prescriptions and primarily refers to psychotropic drugs — tranquillisers, anti-depressants and hypnotics. The long-term use of these drugs is probably valueless in pharmaceutical terms as patients become resistant to their effects and habituated, or worse addicted, to taking them. The drugs themselves are often expensive and the doctor/patient agreement to prescribe them is the relationship referred to by Balint where it is more comfortable to both

parties to maintain the *status quo* rather than change it.
(iv) Those medications in the 'fringe' group. This includes cough medicines and antibiotics prescribed for doubtful reasons without an assessment of the patient's need. If the patient feels that he requires a cough medicine then a practice policy directed towards encouraging him or her to purchase a proprietary brand will save a considerable amount of practice time, and the DHSS a great deal of money! A case can rarely be made for repeat prescribing of antibiotics without an assessment of the patient, except for those patients with chronic bronchitis or on long-term treatment for chronic urinary tract infection.

The system itself must meet the following requirements:

(i) Be simple, cheap and easy to administer.
(ii) The record should show what drugs were last prescribed and when.
(iii) The patient should understand how the system operates and be able to obtain the request within 24 hours but not expect it almost instantaneously.
(iv) There should be an inbuilt method of measuring the patient's request against the drug supplied so that an idea can be obtained of the patient's compliance with instructions.
(v) The system should incorporate some method of feeding back to the doctor information about his pattern of prescribing.

The importance of an efficient repeat prescribing system really sums up the value of having efficient records for all aspects of practice work.

In Summary

A good record system will enable a general practitioner to feel that he or she is in command of his or her workload rather than be overwhelmed by it. This chapter has described the essential features of medical records and registers in general practice. An extended discussion of these and other systems will be found in Chapter 22.

References and Further Reading

Dawes, K.S. 'Survey of General Practitioner Records', *British Medical Journal*, 3 (1972), pp. 219-23.

Eimerl, T.S. & Laidlaw, A.S. *A Handbook for Research in General Practice*, 2nd edition (Edinburgh and London: E. & S. Livingstone, 1969).

Elliot, A., Valdez, N., Dempsey, C. & Cooper, P. 'Art Evaluation of the A4 Folder System in General Practice', *Journal of the Royal College of General Practitioners*, 29 (1979), pp. 85-9.

Hawkey, J.K., Loudon, I.S.L., Greenhalgh, G.P. & Bungay, G.T. 'New Record Folder for Use in General Practice', *British Medical Journal*, 4 (1971), pp. 667-70.

Howie, J.G.R. *Research in General Practice* (London: Croom Helm, 1979).

Loudon, I.S.L., 'Record-Keeping in General Practice', *Update*, 10 (1975), pp. 259-67.

Maycock, C. 'G.P. records: Paediatric Development Card', *British Medical Journal*, 2 (1979), pp. 1453-4.

Pinsent, R.F.J.H. 'The Evolving Age-Sex Register', *Journal of the Royal College of General Practitioners*, 16 (1968), pp. 127-34.

Tait, I.G. 'The Clinical Record in British General Practice', *British Medical Journal*, 2 (1977), pp. 683-8.

Weed, L. *Medical Records, Medical Education and Patient Care* (Cleveland Press of Case Western Reserve University, 1969).

Zander, L., Beresford, S.A.A. & Thomas, P. 'Medical Records in General Practice', *Occasional Paper 5: Journal of the Royal College of General Practitioners* (1978).

Chapter 13: Section 2

Examples of Cards Designed to Fit into Standard Medical Record Envelopes

---

1. Summary Card

(a) Front

SUMMARY CARD

Royal College of General Practitioners

Surname	Christian Names
Date of Birth	N.H.S. No.

YEAR	LIFE HISTORY (BLOCK LETTERS)

FAMILY HISTORY

(b) Back

IMMUNISATIONS

	1	2	3	4
Diphtheria				
Wh. Cough				
Tetanus				
Poliomyelitis				
Smallpox				
B.C.G.				

INFECTIONS

Chickenpox		Wh. Cough	
Measles		Mumps	
Rubella		Scarlet Fever	

	Bl. Group
	Rh
	SENSITIVITIES
	O.S.C.I. (Date)

2. *Drug Treatment Card*

(a) Front

B.D. 3A

DRUG TREATMENT CARD

Surname	Forenames	Date of Birth

DRUG SENSITIVITIES AND PRESCRIBING PROBLEMS

Drug	Nature of Problem	Date if Notified

DRUGS FOR REPEAT PRESCRIPTION

Date Started	No.	Drug and Strength	Dose	Date if Stopped

Record episodic prescriptions over page

(b) Back

EPISODIC PRESCRIPTIONS

Date	Ref.	Drug and Strength	Qty.	Dose

RECORD OF SELF-PRESCRIBED DRUGS

Drug and Strength	Frequency of Use

14 COMPUTERS

When the first edition of this book was being planned the text was based on features common to all practices, such as premises, records, staff, and ways in which they might be managed. Computers rated half a page. For the second edition this was increased to two and a half pages. It is a reflection of the increasing number of practices who already have or who are interested in a practice computer system that a full chapter is now thought to be necessary.

Looked at from the simplest point of view a computer system provides a method of storing information, of producing it again on demand, and of analysing it in ways dictated by the programs available. Information is at present usually put in by using a keyboard, but use of light pens, of touch screens, and of voice recognition to make input easier are either coming into use or are under active development.

Storage of information and of programs is usually on floppy discs (cheaper, relatively small capacity) or on hard discs (more expensive, larger capacity). Information is usually produced by the computer either on a visual display unit screen or as a printout.

In a medical practice all information currently stored on paper, e.g. the patients' records, repeat prescription cards, claims for items of service, age/sex registers, income received, expenses, textbooks, journals, Mims, can in theory be stored on the computer and regurgitated at any time. In addition, depending on the availability of programs to 'instruct' the computer all this information can be searched and analysed either in part or in whole — and the results made available to the practice. Finally, it is possible to receive information from outside the practice from a variety of sources using telephone lines. Prestel is one such example. There is little doubt that in the near future it will become possible to transfer information from the practice computer to, for example, the FPC, the laboratory or the hospital — a further move towards reducing paper in a practice.

It is for these reasons that we believe the use of computers will change the way in which family medicine is practised. In practices where they have already been installed they have had profound effects on staff and on practice organisation.

When Should a Practice Consider Getting a Computer System?

Practices usually acquire a computer system for one of three reasons, namely, that one of the partners is enthusiastic, that the practice has an organisational problem, or that the practice is offered a cut-price system.

1. Enthusiasts

Until recently the commonest way for a computer to be introduced into a practice has been through the enthusiasm of one doctor. Such enthusiasts have either bought early samples of general practice systems and have experimented with their use or have bought cheap microcomputers and programmed them themselves or employed people to do it for them. This approach has resulted in significant advances but there have been some unfortunate results, such as loss of records or souring of relationships within a practice. Introduction by an enthusiast is less likely to cause chaos if the practice has been properly prepared (Pringle *et al.*, 1982), if the enthusiast sticks to his own patients and the partners are subsequently persuaded by his success, or if all agree that a computer is the best solution to a practice problem.

2. Practice Problems

There are occasions when a practitioner looks at what is happening in the practice and finds all is not well. It may be that the appointment system is a mess, or that only 20 per cent of registered children are receiving their pre-school boosters, or there is no way of telling whether the records of recently registered patients have been received in the practice or have been misfiled.

From the management angle it is necessary first to find out what is happening, then to look at various ways in which the problem can be resolved. Among possible remedies would be the tightening up of present procedures, changes in the system, institution of a new manual system, or use of a computer. A repeat prescription system is a good example. It might be that agreement by the doctors to sign 'scripts at a different time of day would be all that was needed to improve efficiency, or that a record should be kept of drugs requested and issued, or that a computer system should be used to reduce the enormous amount of staff time committed to producing repeat prescriptions.

3. A Cut-price System

Companies who are developing computer systems for general practice always wish to get as near to reality as possible, testing their systems under a full practice workload and developing programs which will be of practical use. Offers of systems at reduced prices have been and are being made to practices in exchange for the practice providing facilities for testing and developing. Sometimes this arrangement works well. On other occasions practices accepting these offers have become disillusioned at the amount of work they and their staff have put in, often with disruption of routines, without receiving practical benefit. Practices should be aware of the hassle which can arise in a development practice and look carefully at such offers.

In summary, we do not advise that a practice should invest in a computer system unless they have considered carefully the functions which the system will carry out and the reasons for choosing a computer rather than a manual system. The doctors and staff should also be aware of what the introduction of a computer is likely to do to them (see pp. 151-2). In our view a practice should cross these bridges before seriously considering purchase.

Choosing a Computer System

The process of choosing a computer can be complex. Insecure in computer jargon, unsure of the uses to which the system will be put, confused by computer salesmen, a choice may easily be made which is later regretted. It is helpful to consider the question under the following headings:

1. What Do You Want Done?

This decision will involve looking at the practice organisation, deciding what task or tasks would benefit from computerisation now, what tasks may or will be added in future. This will determine the facilities needed.

2. Your Practice

The size of the practice, number of patients, quantity of information you normally store about each patient. This together with the number of facilities you need, will determine the amount of memory you require and the sort of backup you use in case of failure.

3. The Way You Plan to Use the System

It may be that the functions you require will involve only one operator in one place, several operators in one place using the same keyboard at different times for different tasks, several operators using different keyboards at different places independently. These decisions whether single user or multiuser, simultaneous or sequential will determine the complexity (and effect the cost) of the system.

4. What Finance is Available

Methods of financing and the total amount available will vary from practice to practice. Decisions have to be made on these matters and whether a lump sum should be found or whether the cost should be spread out over a number of years.

5. What Computer Systems are Available

Having completed these preliminary stages the practice should have a good idea of what it wants within a given price range. The next stage is to match these requirements against the computer systems available. Medical computer magazines in this country (such as *Practice Computing* and *Computer Update*) have articles describing systems and provide addresses of computer companies. The Central Office of Information for General Practice will supply a list of computer systems currently available, together with further information about most of them. It is also important to take into account the contracts each company offers, the backup and maintenance arrangements, and the training offered.

6. Making the Decision

What is needed by the practice and what is available may match. If not, decisions as to whether and to what extent the practice is willing to compromise, have to be made. There are two further factors to be taken into account. Firstly, the decision should be related not just to present need but to the direction and speed in which the organisation of the practice is changing. It is easy to underestimate this factor and practices with computers who have wished to upgrade their systems have sometimes in the past found it impossible to do so. Secondly, the effect of the computer on practice routine should be considered. Some systems and practices mesh in well together. For others the way a particular system carries out a particular task would mean a revolution in practice working methods which might not be very popular.

Finally, one of the most important factors in making the decision is to visit a practice or practices in which the systems under consideration are already installed, and to talk to the partners and staff who operate them. In this way it is possible to see how the system works under a real workload in the real world. Such advice is invaluable. A list of users is held by the Central Information Service at 14 Princes Gate, London (see Appendix: Useful Addresses).

Tasks Commonly Undertaken by Computer systems

Reviews of current applications are available from a number of sources (Jones, 1983; Pringle & Lloyd, 1984).
The two main categories of task are:

1. Storage of Information and Production on Demand

The categories of information usually stored up to now have been concerned with the treatment records of individual patients (with particular emphasis on repeat prescriptions and immunisation states), with clinical records of individual patients (total or summarised, in plain text or coded) and with the names, addresses and other registration details of patients in the practice. A more recent introduction is the storage of 'prompts' to be produced on a certain day or with a certain record.

But it is clear that the above is only a minute proportion of the total information held in the practice in one form or another. There is still some way to go before it can all be stored in such a way that it is available when where and at the speed it is needed.

2. Search and Analysis of Information

It is in this group of tasks that a suitably programmed computer system has the edge over most manual systems. Always provided that the basic information is inserted by the practice, searches and analyses can be made involving one two or more factors. By setting the parameters it is possible for the system to provide, for example, a list of ten-year-old girls registered with the practice who need rubella immunisation (and a list of eleven-year-olds who have slipped through the net). It is possible to obtain names and addresses of patients with diabetes who have not seen the doctor for over a year. It is possible to compare workloads and prescribing habits. Although in most practices the ability to carry out these and other tasks will be used as an 'office aid' in day-to-day practice organisation, there is clearly tremendous potential for use in other ways.

The present position is that commercially available systems do carry out tasks which are relevant to service practices. The extent to which they are shown to be of practical use in the 150 practices involved in the Department of Industry Micros for GPs Scheme will become clear when the results of evaluation of the scheme (Hall, 1983) are published.

Living with a Computer System

Installing a computer and loading it with all the information which the practice considers necessary can be a long and difficult task, especially if the way the information is stored on paper records leaves something to be desired. For successful introduction the aims should be that partners and staff understand what is happening, and that partners and staff maintain motivation during the introductory period.

The following lessons on how to attain these aims have been learnt the hard way by pioneering practices:

1. all partners and involved staff should take part in the discussions and decisions before the computer system arrives.
2. all concerned should be given the opportunity to read relevant articles and to see a system or systems in action.
3. discussions should cover:
   the way that the present manual systems run and changes necessary with the introduction of the computer;
   should manual systems be superceded, be phased out or run parallel;
   methods of loading the computer (by whom, when);
   first use of the computer (what information to be loaded first);

verification or not of the accuracy of information being loaded.

4. The early production of a defined output (such as repeat prescriptions) which lessens a repetitive chore is greatly appreciated.

5. once the system has been introduced it should take its place as a normal part of the organisation, keeping a low profile and becoming generally accepted.

6. extension of use of the computer should await successful completion of previous stages.

There is no doubt that living with an established computer system presents few problems and will become commonplace. Its introduction, however, can be a traumatic event and should be approached with due appreciation of the difficulties which may be encountered.

Further Reading

Computers in Primary Care. Occasional Paper 13, Royal College of General Practitioners (London, 1980).

Hall, M.S. *'Micros for GPs', The Royal College of General Practitioners Members Reference Book 1983,* pp. 403-7.

Jones, R.V.H. 'Computing in General Practice', in *Medical Annual 1983* (Bristol: John Wright and Sons, 1983).

Pringle, M. Dennis, J. and Hutton, A., 'Computerization — the choice', in *British Medical Journal,* 284 (1982), pp. 165-8.

Pringle, M. and Lloyd, R., *Computers in General Practice,* in press (Oxford: OUP).

Chapter 14: Section 2

A. Checklist of points to consider when a practice is contemplating the purchase of a computer

Practice decisions

1. Why do we want a computer?
2. What do we want it to do?
3. Who will use it, how many people, how many terminals?
4. How much memory do we need?
5. How fast a printer do we need?

6. Where will it go, bearing in mind space needed, heat generated, noise generated, electrical supply?
7. How much money can we afford?

Computer Decisions

1. What systems are available to provide the functions we need within the price range we can afford?
2. Is the system expandable?
3. What is the reputation of the company for
   — system reliability
   — system maintenance
   — upgrading of programs and production of new programs
   — responsiveness to the needs and problems of their customers
   — documentation of their system
   — training in the use of their systems

B. Technical Points

1. Memory: for an 'average record' (i.e. registration details and a full summary) allow a minimum of one K (kilobyte) per patient which equals 1 megabyte per 1,000 patients. Remember that on hard discs one or several sections of the disc will be occupied by programs.
Floppy discs: the storage capacities are constantly rising. At present one 5½" double sided double density floppy disc commonly holds 500K on each side, i.e. enough space for up to 1,000 patient records on a disc.
Hard discs: common sizes are 5 megabyte, 10-12 megabyte, 18 megabyte and 30 megabytes.

2. Printers: Dot matrix printers are faster but produce less legible output. The speed is usually between 60-160 letters (characters) per second.
Daisy wheel printers produce higher quality print (typewriter quality) but are slower, about 17-40 letters per second and more expensive.

C. Help

Sources of help include:

1. Central Information Services (see Appendix II: Useful Addresses) who will provide particulars of systems available and a list of computer users.
2. *Practice Computing* and *Computer Update* are regular publications which provide useful reviews and articles.
3. Colleagues: the most effective way of finding out how well a particular computer works in practice is to visit a colleague who has one.
4. The British Primary Health Care Specialist group of the British Computer Society produces a newsletter for members and arranges meetings and symposia. The membership secretary is Hugh Fisher, Manager, Exeter FPS Computer Unit, Bowmoor Annexe, Royal Devon & Exeter Hospital (Wonford), Barrack Road, Exeter EX2 5DW.

15 AUDIT — WHAT'S HAPPENING

Of the adjectives applied to general practitioners the word 'busy' is one of the most common. Many patients and many doctors visualise general practitioners as being almost under siege, confronted with a vast number of patients constantly and simultaneously wanting to see them, and living in a precarious state of balance in which the doctor's supply of time barely meets the demands made upon it.

There are good historical reasons for this image. The most obvious is that with the introduction of the National Health Service in 1948 it was accepted in a Western society for the first time that open access to general medical care should be available for the whole population of a country on a continuing basis day and night throughout the year. Certainly at that time doctors were fearful that, given a completely free service without any direct financial involvement by the patient, they would face impossible demands and might not be able to meet all the requests that they received.

Furthermore, at that time a large number of general practitioners were practising single-handed. By today's standards their administrative support was rudimentary. Most did not have a secretary or a receptionist, and many relied on their wives and families for help.

It is hardly surprising that the image of the 'busy' doctor arose although few general practitioners could define accurately the amount of work they were doing.

Recognition that unless a general practitioner can analyse what is going on within the practice he is unlikely to be able to make reasoned changes to improve its efficiency has been slow in gaining general acceptance.

Organisational Revolution

In the 1950s, pioneered largely by the Royal College of General Practitioners, a variety of aids to practice organisation were introduced. The employment of secretaries using typewriters and dictaphones was encouraged. A variety of new ways of organising and abstracting records was introduced, of which age/sex registers (introduced by the Birmingham Research Unit of the College) and the diagnostic register originally called the 'E' book (introduced by Dr. T.S. Eimerl) were among the most important.

About the same time a growing number of general practitioners began to analyse their own work and to keep records of the number of consultations and home visits they were doing. The introduction of appointment systems helped them to analyse their own workload and provided a baseline for comparisons of the amount, type and range of work carried out.

At first it was mainly the enthusiasts and research workers in general practice, a tiny minority of general practitioners as a whole, who were most interested. However, as time went on and reports such as the *Present State and Future Needs* of the Royal College of General Practitioners appeared, more general practitioners found it interesting to be able to compare their workload with that of their colleagues and to learn about new ideas of organisation from them. A study of the journals of general practice in the 1950s shows a large number of articles reporting appointment systems and workload studies in different type of practices.

During the 1960s and 1970s these ideas spread. They ceased to be the prerogative of a small minority but became common practice of first hundreds and then thousands of general practitioners. Nowadays, indeed, it is expected that all training practices will have age/sex registers and will be able to demonstrate their use to the vocational trainees (*Journal of the Royal College of General Practitioners,* 1977). Similarly, the number of practices which are able to analyse consultations by diagnosis and which have lists of patients with various chronically handicapping conditions is growing all the time.

Since all these systems cost both time and money and involve general practitioners in additional work the questions are bound to be asked, 'What is their purpose? What is their value? How can they help me in running my practice?'

Advantages

The advantages to general practitioners of knowing what is going on in their practices can be considered under four main headings:

(1) Practice management and planning

(2) Clinical standards
(3) Improving income
(4) Professional morale.

1. Practice Management

General practitioners have to take decisions about a whole variety of problems, both clinical and management. All general practitioners are daily brought into contact with clinical problems but until recently the nature of management problems and the influence they had on clinical matters were largely unrecognised.

General practitioners have to take decisions about the number of staff to employ, their qualifications, their duties, and the degree of responsibility which can appropriately be delegated to them. They have to decide whether or not to have an appointment system. If there is an appointment system how many patients should be booked each hour? They have to decide whether or not their appointment system is working satisfactorily.

There are three considerations which in our view make the gathering of management information and feedback essential:

(a) Decision-taking should be based on fact.

It is obvious that the ability to take such decisions must depend upon the information available to the decision-maker. Yet paradoxically, because of its history, general practice has grown up in a tradition of decision-taking by hunch, often without the benefit of (and sometimes in the face of) facts.

Almost all studies of decision-taking in industrial organisations emphasise the importance of rational thinking in the light of fact. One of the main advantages of regular documentation of various practice activities such as the number of consultations, and the number of patients seen by each doctor, is that the general practitioner partners who, as was shown in Chapter 7, are the apex of the decision-taking process, are better informed and therefore likely to take better decisions. Put another way, without some form of feedback about what is actually happening decisions about systems and staff are taken in the dark.

(b) Basic statistics are necessary for comparison.

An allied and important consideration is that once basic statistics about a practice have been established, such as the total number of patients on the lists, their age/sex distribution, and rate of contact with the doctor, it becomes possible to compare the practice with other practices both nationally and regionally. Substantial variation from colleagues is an indication for review which may in itself lead to new ways of solving problems.

(c) Basic statistics can show trends.

Finally, knowing that information is being collected and being able to see it and discuss it over a period of time helps the practice staff morale considerably. It may enable partners to adjust staffing or systems long before outright complaints and grievances occur. For example, in one of our practices a steadily rising quantity of work in the treatment room was shown in the quarterly and annual returns. A decision was therefore taken to increase the number of nursing hours in the practice before grievances arose with the practice nurses.

Vital Statistics

One group of figures is so important that we regard them as 'vital statistics'. We recommend that they should be kept by every general practitioner who works a personal list system and by every group of doctors who do not.

The number of times each patient comes to the surgery on average during the year is known as the *annual consultation rate* and the average number of times each patient is visited at home each year is the *home visiting rate.* The two added together form the total *doctor-patient contact rate.*

If a record is kept of the number of consultations by each doctor's registered patients (or all consultations for a group) and the number of home visits then these three figures can be calculated quite easily. Big changes can occur within a few years. It is only by looking at these statistics that practitioners can define trends so that they may have facts on which to adjust their practice policies.

Example 1: Practice Policies. The following figures were kept for the six consecutive years for the patients registered with one of the authors in a three-partner practice in Exeter. The general trend of both the consultation rate and the home visiting rate (and of the

Table 15.1: Vital Statistics

Year	*Surgery consultation rate per patient per year*	*Home visiting rate per patient per year*	*Total doctor-patient contact rate per year*
1	2.85	0.50	3.35
2	2.79	0.43	3.23
3	2.65	0.35	2.99
4	2.46	0.36	2.82
5	2.68	0.41	3.09
6	2.56	0.33	2.89

total doctor-patient contact rate) is downwards. Furthermore, they show a fall in the home visiting rate per patient of as much as a third in six years.

In this practice over the years in question two policy decisions had been taken by the partners both of which might have caused an increase in the doctor-patient contact rate. In the first place, a policy of encouraging preventive procedures within the practice was increasingly and systematically pursued. In the second, a move was made towards explanation to the patient while reducing the number of prescriptions issued.

In practice it could be demonstrated that neither of these policies had resulted in an increased patient-doctor contact rate. They were therefore continued.

Example 2: Personal Care. When in one practice the partners changed their policy from letting patients see the first doctor available to guiding them to see their own doctor, the question naturally arose — was the policy working? Extraction from the figures over a period of two years showed that the percentage of patients who saw their own doctor rose from 48 at the beginning of the period to 68 at the end. Receptionists as well as doctors found these facts interesting. The measures which had been instituted were judged to be working successfully, and a joint decision was taken to continue.

In the hurly-burly of the day-to-day flow of patients going through a reception desk it is often not possible for the staff to see such broad general trends, and feedback of this kind greatly adds to the interest of their job.

2. *Clinical Standards*

It is increasingly being recognised that clinical standards depend on record-keeping (*Journal of the Royal College of General Practitioners,* 1980). It is difficult for a doctor systematically to organise care for a patient if he has no management plan. The care of a hypertensive patient, for example, depends on blood-pressure readings being recorded at regular intervals. Similarly, the care of patients with asthma increasingly depends on good documentation of serial peak-flow readings. Care of patients with epilepsy depends on a record of fits and effects of treatment. We are all human and without notes we cannot always remember what target result or plan of campaign was agreed with the patient.

If a recorded management plan is necessary for the patient's own doctor it is even more necessary for partners and colleagues in these days of group practice, vocational training, longer holidays and rotas.

One of the great advantages of miniaturisation (Gray, 1978) is that monitoring systems for the chronically handicapped are increasingly coming within the power of general practitioners to control and use. Within the last few years, for example, mini peak-flow meters and portable machines for testing blood sugars have become available at prices most general practices can afford. Thus it becomes possible to monitor asthmatics and diabetics as accurately now as most hospital clinics could do only a few years ago. In this way standards of care can rise quickly and the science of medicine be made available to a much greater number of patients in the population.

Furthermore, once there are good record systems it becomes possible to know what is going on in a whole group of patients with a common condition. Diagnostic registers, for example, make it possible for a general practitioner to identify all his patients with asthma, diabetes, epilepsy or hypertension, and examine the effectiveness of his care.

Such analysis of the clinical record is increasingly being carried out in training practices both by trainers and trainees. The first results are sobering (Kratky, 1977). It is only by examining what we are trying to do and whether we are succeeding that standards can eventually be improved.

3. *Improving Income*

General practitioners are independent contractors (Chapter 2). A proportion of their income depends on item-of-service fees for preventive medicine. In Britain the average income of general practitioners from these fees is only about 7 per cent of the total NHS income (Chapter 17), whereas in some of the authors' practices much higher fees are currently being obtained.

For example, in one of our practices with three partners, a total list size of 6,639 patients, and an age-sex structure approximating to the national average, the item-of-service fees for the quarter ending 31 March 1980 were as follows:

	£	*Annual equivalent (£)*
Maternity medical services	711	2,844
Contraceptive care	656	2,624
Immunisations	624	2,496
Cervical cytology tests	197	788
Night visits	101	404
Emergency treatment	27	108
Dental haemorrhage	0	0
	£2,316	£9,264 p.a.

In this practice the total percentage of item-of-service fees as a proportion of NHS practice income at 31 March 1980 was 17.6 per cent. On analysing why this practice can have two and a half times the amount of income from item-of-service fees as the national average, it appears that the income depends on the systems which were set up to enable the partners to know what was going on in the practice.

Example 3: Cervical Cytology. When the partners reviewed the current regulations governing NHS payments for cervical cytology (Red Book, Statement of Fees and Allowances, para. 28.1), it immediately became clear that some of the partners were not familiar with the regulations and on relatively few occasions were claiming the appropriate fee on Form FP74. There was unanimous agreement to start increasing the practice income from this source with the results shown in Table 15.2. These figures show a fourfold increase in practice income for cervical cytology over a two-year period. In other words, the practice income from cervical cytology fees rose from a rate of £193 a year to a rate of £789 a year within two years.

Table 15.2: Cervical Cytology

Year	Quarter	Quarterly payments for cervical cytology
		Cytology campaign started
1	1	48.30
	2	66.70
	3	62.70
	4	84.70
2	1	72.50
	2	104.40
	3	159.80
	4	102.00
3	1	197.20

Example 4: Tetanus Immunisation. The partners in the same practice read with concern about the death from tetanus of a fit middle-aged man in the United Kingdom in 1979. A sample of the medical records showed that in relatively few cases was the tetanus immunisation status of its adult patients recorded although the proportion of children immunised was high.

The three partners decided to initiate a tetanus preventive campaign by offering patients a tetanus immunisation from the practice nurse when they consulted for other conditions. The increase in workload for the practice sisters in the treatment was immediate and the consequences for the practice income have been considerable, as shown in Table 15.3.

The World Health Organisation advocates that primary care is the natural setting for practical preventive medicine for patients in

Table 15.3: Increased NHS Income after Tetanus Immunization Campaign

Year	Quarter	Practice income from immunisation
1	1	310
	2	274 Income from successive
	3	324 quarters = £1,244
	4	336
		Tetanus immunisation campaign started
2	1	444
	2	609 Income for four successive
	3	543 quarters = £2,219
	4	623

their local communities. The primary health care team, working together closely in general practice, is ideally equipped to bring practical preventive medicine to the vast mass of the population. In the United Kingdom the National Health Service appropriately recognises this responsibility and has provided several financial incentives to undertake it.

That such preventive medicine should be undertaken in general practice is desirable for patients, good for the health of the community and is in the professional interests of the general practitioner and his nursing colleagues who gain in professional satisfaction. Moreover, the practice gains financially.

4. Morale

One of the most important touchstones in determining a doctor's attitude to general practice lies in his attitude to the job itself. In Britain today there are doctors who find general practice tedious, boring, and exasperating, who are out of sympathy with the demands of their patients and see themselves as harried and harassed in their everyday work. Such doctors have low professional morale, and may be heard complaining about their patients, their terms of service and the large amount of trivia in their work.

Side by side with these doctors, sometimes even in the same street, are general practitioners who find general practice intellectually demanding, professionally stimulating and emotionally satisfying. They like their job, are ready and willing to accept the new responsibilities, and are prepared to spend substantial amounts of their free time researching, teaching, or developing their discipline.

It was Irvine in 1978 who first identified these two populations of doctors but subsequently Robinson (1979), a former Chairman of the Patients Association, also commented on them. 'Good practices are getting better so fast that they are almost beyond criticism ... By contrast the rump of the profession, often working in areas with highest morbidity and mortality, looks worse and worse.'

We believe that one of the main differences between these two groups of doctors is that the one accepts life as it comes, and in the absence of information and feedback has no way of making logical changes in the way he organises his practice, whereas the other knows what is going on and can do something logical and practical if things are going wrong. Moreover, in the second group positive encouragement is given to both staff and partners if feedback shows that the practice is working well and that practice policies are proving successful.

The doctor no longer feels a helpless prisoner of forces beyond his or her control. It is our experience that once practices do organise feedback and do know what is going on then professional morale rises dramatically. We have no doubt that information systems, whether they are in organisational, clinical or financial terms are to the benefit of patients, doctors and staff.

To have reached this point in a chapter on audit without having mentioned the word must constitute some sort of record. Audit involves counting and measuring, followed by analysis. This is what this chapter has been all about.

References

Gray, D.J. Pereira. 'General Practitioners and the Independent Contractor Status', *Journal of the Royal College of General Practitioners*, 27 (1977), pp. 750-6.

_____ James Mackenzie Lecture 1977. 'Feeling at Home', *Journal of the Royal College General Practitioners*, 28 (1978), pp. 6-17.

_____ 'The Key to Personal Care', *Journal of the Royal College of General Practitioners*, 29 (1979), pp. 666-78.

Irvine, D.H. 'The Future of the College', *Journal of the Royal College of General Practitioners*, 28 (1978), pp. 146-53.

Journal of the Royal College of General Practitioners. Editorial, Age-sex Registers, 27 (1977), pp. 515-17.

_____ Editorial, Systematic Surveillance, 30 (1980), p. 2.

Kratky, A.P. 'An Audit of the Care of Diabetics in One General Practice', *Journal of the Royal College of General Practitioners*, 27 (1977), pp. 536-43.

National Health Service (Family Practitioner Services), *Statement of Fees and Allowances Payable to General Medical Practitioners, The Red Book* (London: DHSS, n.d.)

Robinson, J. *The Lancet*, 2 (1979), p. 211.

Royal College of General Practitioners. *Present State and Future Needs of General Practice.* Reports from General Practice No. 16 (London: *Journal of the Royal College of General Practitioners*, 1973 and 1976).

PART FIVE:

MONEY

16 THE RED BOOK

It is easy to write that 'the fees and allowances payable to general medical practitioners in England and Wales who are in contract with Family Practitioner Committees are described in the Red Book'. It is more difficult to persuade doctors of the importance of knowing their way around and of understanding the Red Book. There are disincentives. The language is stilted and tortuous. The matter is detailed and complex. It could never be described as a 'racy read'. But unless a practitioner is aware of his entitlements practice income suffers. Both the services which he can offer to his patients and his take home pay may be affected. There are, for instance, practices we have visited who do not think they can afford to buy peak flow meters or books on general practice or an ECG machine, but who at the same time are unaware of the advantages of taking advanced payment for 'leave' (para 12.5) and 'on account' (paras 76.1-3), of the difference between payments for emergency treatment (paras 33.1-6) and temporary residents (paras 32.1-8), or of the significance of paragraph 44.5. So we make no apology for using the first chapter in the finance section to set out an analysis and summary of the Red Book.

As this chapter has been designed to be used as a practice guide the text is arranged under topic headings. If a practitioner or member of staff looks up a particular topic under the appropriate heading they will find a resumé of the information which is contained in the numbered paragraphs of the Red Book. In Section 2 of this chapter the contents of the Red Book as at 1984 are listed for cross reference.

The main topic headings used are premises, staff, time off, trainees and trainers fees and allowances, followed by a description of how amendments are negotiated.

Premises

1. *Reimbursement of Rent and Rates*

Eligibility of premises: paras 51.1-51.11

These paragraphs define the criteria which doctors and premises have to meet before they are accepted for reimbursement.

Payment of rents: Para 51.12a

Rents are paid under three headings, viz. *cost rents* for new purpose-built premises or their equivalent (paras 51.50-51.58), *notional* rents for owner-occupiers (paras 51.22 and 51.24-25), and *economic* rents for premises rented either from local authorities (i.e. health centres, paras 51.59-60) or individuals/companies (paras 51.20-21, 51.27-28).

The term 'current market rent' (paras 51.20, 51.22, 51.25, 51.41, 51.52) may confuse practitioners. It is defined as the rent which the District Valuer judges the premises would attract on the open market in current conditions. Notional and economic rents are based on this assessment.

Payment of rates: para 51.12b, c

These paragraphs describe the types of rates which are reimbursed. General, water and sewage rates are covered.

Reduction of payment: paras 51.15-51.17

Reimbursement may be reduced because private work is carried out in the premises, because part of the accommodation is let out, or because the practice has an interest-free loan under the Group Practice Loans Scheme.

Claims for payment: paras 51.30-51.37

Forms Prem I (notification of details of premises) and Prem II (annual or amending), together with the procedure which follows when these forms are received by the FPC, are described.

Review of rents: paras 51.38-51.49

Reassessment of rents may be made at 3-yearly intervals. The procedure to revise a notional rent or economic rent to the current market rent is described.

Procedure for health centre practices: paras 53.1-53.8

These paragraphs describe the way practitioners in health centres should approach changes for accommodation and contributions in lieu of rates.

Appeals

against non-acceptance of premises: para 51.6

against level of reimbursement: para 51.35

against cost rents: paras 51.58.22-23.

When considering appeals against levels of reimbursement, particularly for notional, economic or current market rents, practitioners have been strongly advised by the General Medical Services Committee to use the services of a qualified surveyor and valuation expert if they decide to appeal. The GMSC holds a list of approved surveyors.

2. *Building and Improving Premises*

NEW separate purpose built premises

Definition

General information

Specific information

Information over procedures to be followed are contained in this section which describes and defines the separate stages which have to be undertaken. This page and a half is essential reading for those undertaking new building and should be available for constant reference.

Variations of the cost rent schemes

includes the following:

renting new premises from a third party: paras 51.54.1,
51.58 14-18

purchase and lease from the GPFC: paras 51.58 1-4
51.58 7-13
51.58 19-21

Accommodation size/standards: paras 51.51
51.52 10-15
51 schedule 1
51 schedule 1

These paragraphs define the maximum size of rooms and circulation space allowed under the scheme for different sized practices, together with what are described as 'desirable features' of the proposed accommodation.

Calculation of interim and final cost rents: paras 51.51
51.52.17
51.53.1

These paragraphs describe the basis on which cost rent payments are calculated by the FPC.

Premises bought for substantial modification

In general the arrangements are very similar to those pertaining to newly-built premises.

Definition of 'substantial modification': para 51.51

Procedures to be followed: paras 51.55 1-2

Substantial modification of existing practice premises

Again the procedures are broadly similar to those for new premises.

Owned by the practice: paras 51.56 1-2
Rented by the practice: para 51.57
Improvements to existing practice premises
eligibility: paras 56.1-6
application for grants: paras 56.9-17
appeals: para 56.18
This section describes the grants which may be available to practitioners for projects to which the cost rent scheme does not apply and for which tax allowances cannot be claimed.

Staff

1. Directly Employed Staff

The following paragraphs are concerned with reimbursements for ancillary staff directly employed by a general practitioner whether he practices in a health centre, in premises rented from a private landlord or in premises owned by the practice.

Eligibility of doctors: para 52.4
Categories of staff to whom scheme applies: paras 52.5-6
Reimbursable hours: para 52.7
These sections lay down the types of staff for whom reimbursement can be claimed, the number of hours claimable per principal (currently 72 hours) and the fact that if a doctor receives less than the full basic practice allowance he/she will only be entitled to claim for one full-time staff or equivalent.
Payments made: paras 52.8-12
Details of the payments which can be made are given in these paragraphs, including the percentage of the staff salary, qualifying superannuation contributions, the employers National Insurance contribution and the percentage of the cost of staff training. Also included are the arrangements made under the scheme for paid holidays, sick leave, and maternity leave.
Claims for payment: paras 52.13-18
Practitioners should particularly note the arrangement which can be made for monthly advances on account for staff payments (para 52.15).
Redundancy payments: para 52.18
Related ancillary staff: paras 52.28-44
Within this section the rules concerning reimbursement of

relatives who are directly employed by the doctor are spelt out. The current allowance is noted in paragraph 1/schedule 1. Claims are made to the FPC on special forms (RAN 1/1A, 2/A and 3).

2. *Staff Not Directly Employed by the Doctor:* para 52.19-26

Certain staff may 'perform qualifying duties' for the practitioner although not directly employed by him/her. In these paragraphs the arrangements for shared time are set out and the criteria which have to be met.

Time Off

Leave payment: para 12.5

The conditions under which part of the total basic practice allowance may be taken to coincide with a holiday or study leave are described.

Prolonged study leave: paras 50.1-12

For study leave lasting between 10 weeks and 12 months certain allowances are available to doctors who plan a course of study which 'is in the interests of medicine in a broad sense or otherwise in the interests of the National Health Service as a whole'.

Sickness and confinement

sickness: paras 481.1-23
sickness of assistants: paras 48.24-27
confinement: paras 49.1-18

If a locum or deputy is employed in case of sickness, practitioners may be entitled to some reimbursement, the amount depending on the length of time he/she has worked in the Health Service, the availability or not of partners, and the length of time the 'incapacity' lasts.

Trainees and Trainers

1. *Trainee Practitioners*

Calculation of salary: para 38.6e I-V

These paragraphs describe the way a trainee's salary is calculated, with information about London Weighting, hospital locum service prior to starting a trainee appointment, incremental progression and premature termination of contract.

Reimbursement of expenses

Removal expenses: paras 38.7-38.10, para 38.12

Trainees are entitled to reimbursement of removal expenses if they necessarily change their accommodation when moving from a NHS post to a practice or from one training practice to another. Reimbursement may cover not only removal of furniture and effects but may include storage, insurance, legal and estate agent fees, other fees involved in house purchase or sale, bridging loans, tenancy agreements. Trainees who are not eligible for normal removal expenses may be able to claim 'miscellaneous expenses grant' (para 38.12) if they are moving into new accommodation. This grant includes such diverse items as 'connection of cooker', 'redirection of mail' and 'tuning of piano'.

Removal losses: para 38.11.d, 38.11.e, 38.13

If by moving to a training post loss is incurred by giving up a rail or bus season ticket, a loss is made on a child's school fees or there are lodging costs of a child left behind for education reasons, these losses may be recoverable. Reimbursement of loss also covers what is described as a 'continuing commitments allowance' (e.g. for a rent and rates contract in the area of previous employment).

Travelling expenses: paras 38.11 a-c, fii-iii, 38.16, 38.24

A trainee may incur travelling expenses when looking for accommodation, on moving to new accommodation, on travelling between permanent accommodation and workplace, or on attending for interview. The extent to which these expenses are reimbursable is described in the above paragraphs.

On call expenses: para 38.17

Reimbursement of lodging expenses when a trainee is on call in a practice at a distance from his permanent home may be reimbursable.

Examination expenses: para 38.43

Travelling and subsistence expenses incurred when sitting postgraduate examination (but not the fees) may be allowed: claim forms GPCF3 from the Family Practitioners Committee.

Miscellaneous allowances: para 38.18

In addition to the 'continuing committment allowance' (q.v.)

a trainee may be eligible for an excess rent allowance as arrangements similar to those for hospital doctors.

Sick pay: paras 38.25, 38.26, 38.27

The arrangements when a trainee is absent because of sickness are described under these paragraphs. There are different arrangements for absence up to two weeks, for two weeks to three months and a period lasting longer than three months.

Maternity leave: paras 38.28 to 38.42

The qualifying conditions, salaries to be paid, arrangements when a trainee fails to return to work, extension of traineeship and other matters pertaining to maternity leave are described.

2. Trainers

Approval of trainers: paras 38.1 to 38.4

The approval of trainers is the responsibility of the General Practice Subcommittee of the appropriate Regional Postgraduate Education Committee. These paragraphs describe the process of approval and the appeals machinery.

Payment of trainers

conditions of payment: para 38.5
rates of payment: para 38.6

These paragraphs describe the various conditions which have to be met by a trainer, and the payments to which he is entitled.

Fees and Allowances

The level of current fees and allowances is shown in para 1 schedule 1 at the beginning of the Red Book. The first part of the book consists of definition of these fees and allowances, conditions under which they are paid and methods of claiming. Headings for the different types of payment are given in Section 2 of this chapter.

Amendments to the Red Book

Alteration of the Schedules of the NHS Regulations is by Act of

Parliament. Alteration to the fees and allowances payable to practitioners are made by negotiation between the profession and the DHSS or following recommendations of the Review Body (see below). Amendments to the Red Book describing the agreed alterations are published as numbered pamphlets entitled SFA, e.g. SFA99 was published in September 1983. SFA stands in this instance for 'Statement of Fees and Allowances'. These pamphlets are issued by FPCs to all appointed general practitioners and trainees in general practice.

The Review Body itself was set up following the recommendations of the Royal Commission on Doctors' and Dentists' Remuneration in 1960. The main aim was to avoid recurrent disputes about remuneration by establishing an impartial body which would recommend just levels of payment after hearing evidence from both the government and the profession. The Review Body is free to obtain additional information from whatever source it wishes. It is free to decide its own methods of work, the periods that its recommendations should cover, and how often to undertake reviews. There are seven members and a chairman. In practice in each of the past six years there has been one main review in the spring supplemented by interim reviews when the need arose.

In addition to this formal review machinery, direct negotiations between the profession and the Department of Health and Social Security occur at regular monthly meetings. The general practitioners who negotiate on behalf of the profession are appointed annually by the General Medical Services Committee from among its members. The GMSC currently (1984) has 80 members composed of elected and appointed representatives. The majority of members (42) are general practitioners who are elected by Local Medical Committees throughout the country. A further six are elected annually by the conference of Representatives of Local Medical Committees.

Local Medical Committees in turn are composed of general practitioners, each of whom has been elected by fellow practitioners in his practice district. So when it negotiates with the government on terms and conditions of service the General Medical Services Committee represents the interests of every general practitioner in the country, whether or not he be a member of the BMA, RCGP, MPU or any other organisation. Because the BMA is the only negotiating body for general practitioners recognised by the government, however, a typical British compromise has resulted in the GMSC being recognised as a 'craft' committee within the BMA although some of its members may not be members of the Association.

Summary

This chapter has attempted to point out the importance which practitioners should attach to understanding the Red Book and keeping the copies in the practice up to date. It is particularly important that the practice manager or senior secretary should also be involved in this updating in order that he or she may be fully aware of the changes in fees and allowances which may directly affect the practice and its work. We recommend that a partner or member of staff is nominated to insert the new SFA notices as they arrive into the practice copies of the Red Book. This partner or member of staff should draw partners' attention to relevant changes either individually or in a practice meeting.

Chapter 16: Section 2

Contents pages of the Red Book as at November 1984

Statement of Fees and Allowances payable to General Medical Practitioners in England and Wales

CONTENTS

Part I — General

Part II — Payments to Practitioners Providing Unrestricted General Medical Services

Part III — Payments to Practitioners Providing Restricted Services or with Limited Lists

Part IV — Calculation of Lists and Arrangements for Payment

Example of an SFA: SFA 97

In order to keep the Red Book up to date insertion of SFA 97 involved removing old pages 28(b) to 32 inclusive and replacing with new pages marked 29, 30, 31, 32 and 33 each labelled SFA97. The new pages arrived at all practices together with a notice as follows:

NATIONAL HEALTH SERVICE

GENERAL MEDICAL SERVICES

AMENDMENTS TO STATEMENT OF FEES AND ALLOWANCES

1. The Secretary of State has made a determination in accordance with Regulation 24 of the National Health Service (General Medical and Pharmaceutical Services) Regulations 1974 and has amended the Statement of Fees and Allowances as set out in the attached pages. The Secretary of State has consulted the representatives of the profession in accordance with Regulation 24.
2. Any question arising out of this SFA should be addressed to the Family Practitioner Committee.

EXPLANATORY NOTE
(This note does not form part of the Statement of Fees and Allowances)

Paragraph 27/Schedule 1, item 7, of the Statement of Fees and allowances was amended with effect from 1 September 1981 so that the vaccination against rubella of girls between their 10th and 14th birthdays now attracts the appropriate fee. Item 1 of Schedule 1 was amended with effect from 6 September 1982 so that the vaccination against whooping cough of children before the age of 6 now attracts the appropriate fee.
These amendments to the Statement were announced in HN (FP)(81)34/FPN 293 and HN(FP)(82)22/FPN 319 respectively and, in accordance with those circulars, pages 30 and 32 of the Statement have now been reprinted.
September 1983

N.B.: The importance of this SFA for practice organisation is that it notified the fact that the age for which fees could be claimed for immunising girls against rubella had been lowered from 11 years to 10 years.

17 FINANCE: MONEY IN

It is only comparatively recently, since family doctors began to organise themselves into larger groups and partnerships, that the importance of having clear and accurate financial accounts has been generally appreciated. Larger practices result in more complex organisation, higher shared income and higher shared expenses. It is important for the partnership that each partner should have a clear idea of where the money comes from and where the money goes. In this chapter possible sources of practice income are discussed. In Chapter 18 the subject of practice expenses is considered.

General practitioners have three types of income:

(1) Personal income from sources other than medical practice.
(2) Private income from medical work outside the National Health Service.
(3) Income from the National Health Service.

The 'practice income' of a general practitioner, whether he is in partnership or in single-handed practice, consists of income from the medical work undertaken in 'practice time'.

1. Personal Income

This is unconnected with the practice and does not usually involve partners. For most such income (e.g. interest from stocks or shares owned personally by the general practitioner) poses no problem of definition. There may be, however, some difficulty in deciding whether income from such activities as writing or lecturing is 'personal' or has taken place in 'practice time' and should therefore be classed as practice income. This is a matter which should be covered in the partnership agreement.

2a. Private Income for Most General Practitioners

1. Insurance Examinations and Reports

Medical reports are used by insurance companies to assess the risk (and therefore the premium) for life and sickness insurance policies. These reports may either be full reports involving examination of the patient, or short reports on the medical history of the patient culled from the practitioner's knowledge and the medical record. For some general practitioners who are medical examiners for large insurance companies, these examinations may form a considerable proportion of their work. Nevertheless, most general practitioners do some insurance work.

Satisfactory medical reports are also required by insurance companies before they will insure an elderly person to drive a car. Companies vary regarding the age at which they start demanding a medical examination, and the frequency with which this has to be repeated. It is usual for an elderly driver to go to his own general practitioner for this examination but it is quite in order for him to go to any doctor of his choice.

2. *Other Medical Examinations and Certificates*

Medical examinations are required or requested for many other purposes, e.g. when applying for a heavy goods vehicle driving licence, for fitness to take up a job, or to go on a diving course. For all certificates involving a medical examination which are not covered by National Insurance Regulations, the general practitioner is entitled to payment.

Although vaccination and immunisation are procedures to which a patient is entitled under the Health Service, the provision of a certificate stating that these procedures have been carried out also attracts a fee.

3. *Legal Reports*

Most general practitioners will appear in Court as a witness at some time in their professional lives, probably as a witness of fact rather than an expert witness. They will also be required on occasions to give evidence at a Coroner's Court. For these attendances they are entitled to a fee.

In common with any other citizen who may have been involved in such episodes as an assault, car accidents, or drunken brawls, a general practitioner may be asked by the police to provide a report as a witness. For such a report the practitioner is not entitled to a fee. But should a report be requested by the police which involves expression of a medical opinion then a fee should be charged.

Reports made at the request of the police after a doctor has examined someone at a police station fall into this category. In most cities and larger towns these examinations are carried out by the 'police surgeon' (who is usually a local general practitioner), but in country districts there may be no such appointment. If a person who is detained in a police station asks to see his own general practitioner, then that consultation and examination does not fall under the normal terms of service and the practitioner is entitled to a fee.

Solicitors may also ask for reports, usually about a patient who is involved in litigation. The fee for this type of report is not standard but depends upon the complexity of the report and the amount of time the practitioner has to spend on it. As these rates tend to vary, advice concerning the current rate can usually be obtained from the local branch of the Law Society.

4. Cremation Fees

The Brodrick Report, published in 1971, suggested major changes in the procedure to be followed before a body could be cremated. At present, however, the cremation certificate consists of two parts: the first part is signed by the doctor who attended the deceased during their last illness; the second part is signed by an independent practitioner, who cannot be a partner of the doctor who signed the first part and who must have been fully registered for five years. For each part a fee is paid by the executors of the deceased. Usually the undertaker settles this with the doctor on their behalf.

For many of the services referred to above the scale of fees is standard and agreed. The British Medical Association publish a booklet called *Fees for Part-time Medical Services* which is regularly updated. In many practices, however, the scale of fees suggested by the BMA may not be used — some doctors charging patients less than the agreed rate. If this is so, then great care should be taken to write on the notes *exactly* how much has been charged for which service and when, otherwise misunderstandings ensue between patient and doctor and between one partner and another.

2b. Private Income for Some General Practitioners

Many of the medical activities in which general practitioners indulge attract no fee at all. Examples are the lifeboat service, acting as medical officer at various sporting functions, or as adviser to the Red Cross or St. John's Ambulance. But in most practices at least one principal has an outside appointment of some sort. These appointments vary enormously in the responsibilities involved, in the time taken, and in the income received. There are certain broad categories of such appointments and sources of 'private' income.

1. Appointments with Local Authorities

These may be sessional appointments in the medical department for such activities as developmental clinics, or may be appointments to other local authority departments, such as the police or fire brigade.

2. Medical Officers to Schools

Many different types of school have part-time officers who are usually general practitioners. These include boarding-schools, special schools for the handicapped and approved schools. The duties involve not only medical care of individual pupils but also advice to the school authorities on such things as diet, hygiene, and all matters concerning 'public health' in the school setting. Chapter 24 includes further discussion on this subject.

3. Industrial Medical Officers

Large firms employ medical officers as full-time employees, but many medium-sized or small firms employ local general practitioners as part-time advisers. They may be responsible for advising the employer on a prospective employee's fitness for work, on industrial health risks, on general health education matters, and on such matters as the early retirement of employees on grounds of ill-health.

4. Hospital Appointments

Many general practitioners are employed in the hospital service on a sessional basis. Before 1976 the appointment was as a clinical assistant but since that date appointments have also been made to the hospital practitioner grade. Hospital practitioner grade appointments are permanent, but for a job to be so recognised it has to fulfil certain criteria of function and responsibility. The doctor applying for such a post has also to meet certain criteria.

There has been considerable confusion within the profession since this grade was negotiated by the GMSC for general practitioners — and this confusion has not so far (1984) been fully resolved. Until the situation is clarified it is particularly important that a general practitioner applying for a part-time hospital appointment should enquire fully into the terms and circumstances of that appointment.

5. *Appointments to Other Bodies*

Large organisations, such as the Post Office, the IBA, and the BBC, have local part-time medical officers who are usually general practitioners.

6. *Teaching and Lecturing*

Over the past decade there has been a steady increase in the numbers of general practitioners involved in lecturing and teaching. To the staple diet of lectures to the Red Cross or St. John's Ambulance Brigade are now added lectures at postgraduate centres, to medical societies, and to meetings of paramedical workers. There is a growing realisation, both by general practitioners themselves and by other health workers, that general practitioners have unrivalled experience in diagnosis and management at that interface where a person becomes a patient. Although it is probably true to say that few general practitioners find lecturing easy, it is inevitable that the demand for articulate general practitioner lecturers will grow.

7. *Private Patients*

Before 1948 most general practitioners obtained a sizeable proportion of their income from private patients. There were many who had no 'panel patients' and obtained all their income this way. The position is now reversed. There are many practices which do not accept private patients. For those that do, it is usually accepted that the commodity which the private patient buys is convenience rather than quality of medical care. Each general practitioner who does accept private patients should keep a day book. In this the service and the fee to be charged are noted under the appropriate date, so that accounts can be sent out at regular (usually quarterly) intervals.

In some partnerships the proportion of time spent in the practice and the proportion spent on outside appointments varies widely from partner to partner. It is essential for harmony within a partnership that the arrangements for the distribution of this 'private income' are clearly understood from the beginning. It is also essential that when consideration is being given to one partner taking on an additional commitment outside the practice that the implications for all partners are fully discussed and understood.

3. Income from the National Health Service

For the majority of general practitioners, private and personal income is a minor part of the total income. The largest part of most general practitioners' income comes from work done within the Health Service.

As a principal in general practice a doctor is paid by his Family Practitioner Committee under five main headings. In the following section the relevant paragraph number of the Red Book is placed after each category of payment so that reference can be made if more information is needed. The fees and allowances for the current year can also be found in paras 1 and 1/Sch. 1 of the Red Book (see Chapter 16 for further details of this).

1. Fixed Allowances

(a) Basic Allowance (12.1). This is paid to each principal with more than 1,000 patients on his list. A proportion of the allowance is paid to those with less than 1,000 patients. The justification for this payment is that it is to cover the 'expenses of having a practice' but the various expenses have never been specifically named or itemised. It is fair to say that some members of the profession, both in general practice and in the DHSS, regard this as part-salary.

(b) Supplementary Practice Allowance (22.1). This is an extension of the basic practice allowance. It is paid to each general practitioner with more than 1,000 patients on his list who provides an 'out of hours' service (viz. night and weekend cover).

2. Fees Based on Number of Patients

(a) Capitation Fee (21.1). A fee is paid for each patient on the general practitioner's list aged 64 years and under. A slightly higher fee is paid for those aged 65-74, and a higher fee again for those aged over 75.

(b) Supplementary Capitation Fee (23.1). Payment is made to cover the extra work done by a general practitioner for the patient on his list outside 'normal working hours'. There is a capitation payment for the number of patients on his list over 1,000. This is distinct from the night visit fee which is an item-of-service payment.

(c) Temporary Resident's Fee (32.1). This is a fee paid for treating visitors who are in the district for more than 24 hours but less than three months. The rate is lower for a patient who stays less than a fortnight than for one who stays longer. There is a form FP19/EC19 on which this fee is claimed for each temporary resident.

An emergency treatment fee, which currently attracts higher payment than a temporary resident fee, should be claimed for all visitors staying in the district less than 24 hours (para 33.1).

(d) Contraceptive Fee (29.1). This is a fee paid for those patients who sign on for contraceptive services. At present the patient has to sign an annual application for these services (FP1001), which is sent to the Family Practitioner Committee after being countersigned by the doctor to indicate that he has agreed to accept the patient on his contraceptive list. There is a higher rate for fitting an IUD than for general services.

3. Item of Service

Item-of-service fees are paid to the general practitioner for work he does in addition to the general medical care for patients on his list. They are a motley collection; some are paid for preventive measures, such as immunisation, which are blessed by the DHSS (and thereafter called 'public policy'). Others are paid to general practitioners when they perform certain specific (usually unpleasant) duties. Current payments are made for the following services:

(a) vaccination and immunisation (27.1)
(b) cervical cytology (28.1)
(c) night visit fee (24.1)
(d) maternity services and miscarriage (31.1)
(e) arrest of dental haemorrhage (35.1)
(f) emergency treatment fee (33.1)
(g) anaesthetic fee (34.1)

4. Fees Based on a Practitioner's Qualifications

These fees are dependent on either the age, experience, and training of the individual general practitioner, or on his appointment as a general practitioner trainer.

The fees paid for age, experience and training are paid automatically to all who fulfil the criteria. The would-be trainer, however, has to apply to the local Regional Adviser for General Practice for recognition before he is accepted as a trainer. He then has to undergo a selection procedure agreed by the Joint Committee on Postgraduate Training for General Practice. The fees for training are paid to him only for the periods during which he has a trainee.

The references to the fees which are based on practitioners' qualifications are as follows:

(a) vocational training allowance (17.1)
(b) seniority allowance (16.1)
(c) postgraduate training allowance (37.1)
(d) trainer allowance (38.1)

5. Fees for Type or Position of Practice

Practices in different parts of the British Isles may attract payments depending on their location. The additional expense involved for the general practitioner who has a geographically large practice is recognised in rural practice payments.

(a) Rural Practice Payments (43.1). Payments are made to practitioners from a special fund for all those patients who live three miles or more from the main surgery. Most of these payments are made to rural or semi-rural practitioners but those doctors who practise in urban areas may also claim payment if the criteria of the Red Book are met.

Patients attract so many 'units' depending on the distance they live from the main surgery and difficulty of access. Grounds for claiming difficulty of access include narrow roads liable to frequent obstruction (by, for example, livestock, farm vehicles or floods) or the fact that the house cannot be reached by car so that the practitioner can claim 'walking units'. Special arrangements exist for particularly isolated patients, such as those living on small islands.

In all these circumstances it is the doctor who is responsible for claiming the appropriate units from the Family Practitioner Committee. Clearly considerable income may be lost if he does not claim those units to which he is entitled.

(b) Dispensing Fees (44.1). Dispensing doctors have since July 1984 been paid by a drug tariff system similar to that by which chemists are paid. Practitioners who do not normally dispense can claim payment for certain injections and vaccines which they administer personally to patients (44.5). Dispensing practice is discussed further under a separate heading later in this chapter.

(c) Designated Area Allowance (14.1). There are two types of designated area allowance. For type I the area must have been designated for at least three years. For type II, as well as having been designated for at least one year, the average list size in the area must be 3,000 patients or more. Type II attracts a higher allowance.

(d) Initial Practice Allowance (40.1). There are four different types of initial practice allowance labelled A, B, C and D. They are paid to doctors who set up practice in designated areas or in areas where it is agreed by the DHSS and the Medical Practices Committee that a large increase in population may be expected within a few years (such as large housing developments or new towns).

(e) Inducement Allowance (45.1). This is paid as an inducement to maintain a practice in a sparsely populated area, such as the highlands of Scotland.

(f) Group Practice Allowance (15.1). Three or more doctors practising in association (but not necessarily in partnership) may be eligible for a group practice allowance provided the criteria laid down in the Red Book are met.

6. *Reimbursements*

In addition to these direct payments, general practitioners are reimbursed for the rent and rates they pay for their premises, whether these are rents for health centre premises (53.1), privately rented premises, or notional rents for premises which the general practitioners own (51.1). The District Valuer has to inspect the premises and agree an appropriate rent before this reimbursement is made.

Payment is also made for a proportion (currently 70 per cent) of the salary paid to members of the ancillary staff employed by general practitioners, provided that certain conditions are met (52.1), for National Insurance contributions in respect of employed staff (52.8) and for certain staff pension contributions (52.8 and 52.9).

Dispensing Practice

More than 3,000 general practitioners dispense for some or all of their patients. Historically, most doctors provided their patients with advice and medicine. Under the National Health Service the system was continued whereby doctors who had registered patients living more than one mile from the central surgery were able to continue a dispensing service for these patients. For doctors in rural areas, where there was no chemist shop within one mile of the surgery, then all the patients might be on the dispensing list.

It has been argued by the pharmacists that dispensing doctors should have special training. It has also been argued that the existence of dispensing doctors threatens the survival of retail pharmacists in small communities. The Clothier Committee, which was sent up in 1975 to 'find a solution which would secure sensible arrangements for the supply of prescription medicines in rural areas', reported in November 1977. Its main proposal was the establishment of a national statutory body to regulate what was called 'significant changes in dispensing arrangements in rural areas'. The new Rural Dispensing Committee was eventually established in 1983 and with its local counterpart, the FPC's Rural Dispensing Sub-Committee, is attempting to regulate the way in which patients are supplied with medicines. The overriding criterion should be what is best for the patient, but this has to be set against the financial consequences for a dispensing doctor or a pharmacist if a change in practice is allowed. The two professional groups involved have set up compensation funds to help ameliorate the financial effects of any changes agreed.

Method of payment

Until 1 July 1984 the general practitioner who dispenses could do so either under a 'capitation system' or under a 'drug tariff system'.

In practice very few doctors ever chose the former. In June 1984 an amendment to the Red Book (SFA 106) announced the abolition of the capitation system as follows:

1. payment for all dispensing doctors shall be by the drug tariff basis;
2. the reimbursement of basic price (formerly referred to as 'net ingredient cost') shall be abated on the basis of the interim discount scale at Schedule 1;
3. for the calculation of discount all prescriptions shall be submitted in partnership batches;
4. for the calculation of dispensing fees doctors may subdivide partnership batches into individual bundles;
5. VAT reimbursement shall be calculated on the basic price less any discount applicable and on the container allowance;
6. safeguards are introduced to protect doctors unable to obtain discounts because of the remoteness of their practices or the small quantities of drugs they need to supply;
7. all claims shall be submitted direct to the pricing bodies;
8. arrangements for payments for the oxygen therapy service are now at Schedule 3.

The main message of this SFA lay in the first two paragraphs. From 1 July 1984 all dispensing doctors have been paid in a similar manner to retail pharmacists and a scale of abatements was introduced to take into account the fact that most dispensing doctors can get quantity orders at discount.

For each drug they dispense doctors are reimbursed the basic price together with an on-cost allowance (currently 10.5 per cent of the basic cost before discount), a container allowance, a dispensing fee and an allowance in respect of VAT. Retail pharmacists can also claim a broken pack allowance, additional fees for prescriptions which are needed urgently out of hours and are allowed a slightly higher on-cost percentage, but have no superannuation benefits.

Dispensing doctors are normally expected to be able to provide their patients with all required medicines. For these they issue a white prescription form (FP10) which is dispensed from their own dispensary. If for any reason they cannot provide a particular medicine or drug the practitioners may issue a blue FP10 which the patient may take to any retail pharmacist.

At the end of each month the total number of forms collected by the doctors dispensary are sent to the Prescription Pricing Authority for costing and payment.

General Considerations

The dispensing doctor has certain legal obligations. It is his responsibility to see that medicines are dispensed accurately and safely and that all the regulations of the various Drug Acts are conformed with. He may employ a qualified pharmacist who will be entitled to dispense medicines on his own responsibility, but more commonly the dispensing doctor employs a dispensing aide who works under the supervision of the general practitioner. In such circumstances, it goes without saying that the general practitioner is ultimately responsible for medicines dispensed and, in particular, for handling and checking all scheduled and dangerous drugs.

The doctor dispensing medicines is required to collect such prescription charges as may be due from the patient and at the end of each month to forward these moneys to the FPC. Unlike the dispensing chemist these charges are not retained by the doctor and later set against fees and allowances received from the FPC.

In a rural area, the general practitioner frequently has a relatively small list. The dispensing part of the practice may bring in an important proportion of the practice's income. As a rough guide, the 'profit' on dispensing should range from 10-17 per cent of the gross turnover of the dispensary. In part, it would depend on the additional staff costs and the care with which stocks of expensive medicines are controlled.

Patients who are used to the system of receiving a prescription from their doctor and then taking it to a retail chemist for dispensing are often surprised and impressed by the service which patients registered with dispensing practices obtain. Not for them the need to wait to see the doctor and then wait at the chemist's to have their prescription made up, the two operations can be done in the same building usually at the same time. Dispensing doctors, too, have tremendous advantages over their non-dispensing colleagues; during out of hours duty they are able to provide patients with the full course of medicines required and do not have to provide supplies of emergency drugs for which they are not paid. Again, in rural areas, patients are grateful to the doctor who not only visits but at the same time leaves the necessary medicines in the patient's house. Such a service depends on particular circumstances, but often it is extremely satisfying to both doctor and patient.

Dispensing by 'Non-dispensing' Doctors

For general practitioners who do not normally dispense it is possible to make a claim from the FPC on the drug tariff basis for certain vaccines, anaesthetics, injections, sutures and diagnostic reagents which he personally administers to patients. The practitioner buys the drug or reagent, administers it and claims on form FP34 (Doctors). Particulars of the drugs and payments allowed can be found under para 44.5 and para 44 schedules 1-4 in the Red Book.

Influenza vaccine is perhaps the commonest item administered in this way. This provision means that a doctor who carries out minor surgery on his patient can do so at a small cost to the Health Service and with only little cost to themselves. In Section 2 of this chapter a table sets out the typical items used for a minor surgical procedure and the reimbursements made under para 44.5 to a general practitioner who 'dispenses' them himself.

It is worth remembering that all doctors may make use of this regulation and thus reimburse themselves and make a modest profit out of supplying such items.

Method of Payment

The Family Practitioner Committee normally makes payments to general practitioners quarterly in arrears. Any practice can, however, apply to have a proportion of their expected payment made in advance. Many practices have arranged for payment to be made at the end of the first and second months of each quarter, with the balance paid at the end of the quarter. As expenses are incurred and have to be paid throughout the quarter this arrangement has the great advantage of providing cash nearer to the time that the service is provided and the expense incurred.

Average Income

It is extremely difficult to obtain figures reflecting the amount spent on the independent contractor services which are presented

Table 17.1: Average Earnings per Principal, 1982/83

Basic allowances — 21%:	to include
	Basic practice allowance
	Supplementary practice allowance
Capitation fees — 43%:	Regular capitation fees
	Supplementary capitation fees
	Temporary resident fees
	Contraception fees
Item of service — 6%:	Immunisation fees
	Cervical cytology fees
	Maternity fees
	Dental haemorrhage fees
	Anaesthetic fees
	Emergency treatment fees
	Night visit fees
Practitioner qualifications — 10%:	to include
	Designated area allowance
	Initial practice allowance
	Inducement allowance
	Group practice allowance
Reimbursements — 17%:	for premises and staff

in such a way that information useful to general practitioners can be extracted. However, by taking the Review Body figures for 1982/83 and combining them with figures given by the Minister of Health in October 1983 (*Hansard*, 1983) Bowles (1984) has calculated that the average earnings for principals in 1982/83 were as shown in Table 17.1.

Further analysis of the figures reported in *Hansard* showed that the 'average practitioner' carried out the following number of procedures during the year:

Immunisations	217
Contraception registrations	94
Cervical cytology examinations	60
Night visits	23
Temporary resident registrations	
for 15 days	33
for 15 days	22
Emergency treatments	2

The interest of this information for the individual practitioner is that it can be both enlightening and profitable to compare the figures for his practice with the national average. For those areas in which he is below average it may be possible to increase his income with a little planning.

Summing Up

All this may appear very complicated to the new entrant into general practice. These arrangements have been evolved over the years. Each paragraph in the Red Book represents months of negotiation between the profession and the DHSS. There is no doubt, however, that because of a combination of ignorance and idleness, many general practitioners have in the past not received the fees which they have earned.

There are certainly some general practitioners who have not claimed reimbursement of the rent of branch surgeries. There are others who have claimed a temporary resident fee when a larger emergency treatment fee was appropriate. Medical men, and in particular general practitioners, are notoriously careless when it comes to running the business side of their practices. Because so many of us are not temperamentally inclined to 'chase the pennies', one solution is to delegate a senior member of the ancillary staff to scrutinise the amendments to the Red Book (called SFA followed by a number) as they arrive and make sure that the partners are aware of their significance. Another method may be for each partner to take it in turns to be responsible for this.

Whatever method is adopted it is important that the practice is aware of changes which may affect their organisation and practice income.

References

Bowles, R. 'An NHS computer model', personal communication, 1984.
Hansard, 13 October 1983, p. 296.

Chapter 17: Section 2

Example of the Cost of Items used for a minor surgical procedure

		Reimbursed to the doctor by the FPC	
Item used	Cost to the doctor	Reimbursement cost + on cost[a]	Dispensing fee
Xylocaine 1%[b] 1 × 2ml ampoule	13	14.4	59
Suture: sterile, braided† silk BP, Ethicon, W501-one	49	54.1	59
Cost to the doctor	£0.62		
A. Total reimbursed to the doctor			£1.86½
Sterile dressing pack, Drug Tariff[c]	42	X	
Sterile Gauze Pads[c] 8 ply, 1 pack of five	18	X	
Crepe Bandage BPC[c] 7.5cm, one	58p	X	
Melolin PFA non-adherent[c] dressing 1 × 10cm × 10cm	10	X	
B. Cost to doctor of non-reimbursable items	£1.28	X	
NET PROFIT TO DOCTOR	A − B =	£0.58½	

Notes: [a]Each item written on a prescription form FP 10 is reimbursed with an additional 10.5% on cost allowance and a dispensing fee of approximately *59 pence* per item.

[b]Patients do not pay prescription charges for items provided and personally administered by the doctor.

[c]The cost of dressings used may not be reimbursed under paragraph 44.5 but the general practitioner may issue the patient with a prescription for these items before the minor surgical procedure. The patient would thus supply his own dressings. In which case the GP doing this minor surgical procedure would end up with a credit of £1.24½.

18 FINANCE: MONEY OUT

'That's the way the money goes;
Pop goes the weasel.'

The expenses involved in running a practice are of two kinds: running expenses and capital expenses. Capital expenses are defined by accountants as 'all expenditure involved in acquiring fixed assets'. Running expenses, or revenue expenditure, however, are those incurred in 'administering and carrying on the business'. Capital expenditure for general practitioners, therefore, involves the provision of new capital for buying something new, or replacing something which is worn out or outdated. The capital cost is usually written off piecemeal year by year for tax purposes. Running expenses are those which arise from the day-to-day running of the practice. They are set against gross income each year.

With recent changes in the tax laws the difference between these two types of expenses has become more of theoretical than practical importance. However, as most practice accounts are cast in this form, it is important that a young doctor contemplating joining a practice should be able to understand them.

In addition to practice expenses each general practitioner is liable to income tax, National Insurance contributions and superannuation contributions.

Running Expenses

The calculation of running expenses for doctors who work in private premises differs from the calculation for those doctors who work in health centres. In private premises all the expenses are met by the general practitioners themselves. In health centres the cost of running the health centres is initially met by the Area Health Authority which charges the general practitioners using the centre rent and rates for the rooms used and a percentage of the costs of running the centre as a 'service charge'.

A. Practice from Private Premises

The practice expenses of general practitioners who practise from private premises fall into four main categories.

1. Staff Costs

Wages of employed staff
National Insurance contributions for employed staff
Pension contributions for employed staff

The conditions, hours and rates of pay for employed staff are determined by general practitioners themselves. If the staff are not related to the general practitioner or his partners, if they work more than five hours a week, *and* if they perform the qualifying duties laid down in the Red Book (para 52.5), then 70 per cent of their wages will be reimbursed by the FPC up to a total of two full-time (or equivalent part-time) staff for each principal general practitioner who is in receipt of a basic practice allowance, provided that income from private practice is less than 10 per cent of practice income. A form ANC.1 has to be filled in for each qualifying member of staff on appointment and when any change is made in hours employed or wages paid. Claims for reimbursement are made to the FPC each quarter on forms ANC.2 and ANC.3.

National Insurance contributions for employed staff are paid, together with PAYE (Pay As You Earn) income tax deductions from staff salaries, direct to the local tax office each month. The form used and tables to enable the correct amount of PAYE to be calculated are supplied by the local tax office.

National Insurance contributions paid by general practitioners in respect of employed staff are reimbursed in full (52.8). Employers' contributions to certain staff pension schemes are also reimbursed (52.8, 52.9 and a later section in this chapter).

2. Cost of Premises

Rent of premises
Rates for premises
Repairs and redecorations
Insurance of premises

For premises rented from a private landlord, reimbursement of the rent is made by the Family Practitioner Committee provided that the District Valuer considers that the rent charged is appropriate. For premises owned by the partnership as a whole, or by one of the partners, a 'notional rent' based on the current market rent as assessed by the District Valuer is paid. It may be a lengthy process for the practice and the District Valuer to agree an appropriate rent, but practitioners should continue the battle, by appeal if necessary, until a figure which they consider reasonable is obtained. An under-payment of £500 per year amounts to £5,000 in ten years. In case of difficulty advice may be sought from local colleagues and from the secretariat of the General Medical Services Committee through the local member.

Application for reimbursement of rent starts with a description of the premises on a form PREM.1 provided by the FPC. Thereafter quarterly payments are made by the FPC.

The rates for premises used by the practice have to be paid to the local council (as in any other business). Reimbursement of general and water rates (since April 1978) is made by the FPC when they receive evidence that they have been paid.

Redecorations and repairs cover the expenses involved in keeping the paintwork, furniture and fittings up to standard. The usual division of responsibility (which should be laid down in the lease) is that the landlord pays for external and structural repairs, while the practice is responsible for interior repairs and redecoration.

Insurance of premises and contents is the responsibility of the partners. As in any other property insurance a regular review is necessary to make sure that the insurance matches current value. Many partnerships also include insurance for consequential loss incurred in the event of fire or other disaster. Some include life or sickness policies on the partners' lives.

3. Servicing Costs

Telephones
Heat and light
Postage, stationery, printing

These are inevitable costs and may be small or large depending on the amount of thought that has been put into the planning, the standards selected, and the extravagance or care with which the services are used.

4. Professional Costs

Accountancy
Legal costs

Bank charges
Subscriptions
Professional insurance
Books and Journals.

There are few general practitioners who understand the mysteries of accountancy, and there are few accountants who are experts in the intricacies of general practice finance. The process of mutual enlightenment proceeds slowly. Meanwhile the fees paid to an accountant who is versed in medical matters are often more than recovered by him annually through income tax saved.

Bank charges for practice overdrafts, unlike charges for private overdrafts, are allowed against tax and are considered in the income tax section.

Subscriptions to professional societies, such as the BMA or RCGP, may by partnership agreement be paid through the practice account, or may be paid by the individual doctor concerned. There is also an annual retention fee payable to the General Medical Council for retention of the practitioner's name on the Register.

Insurance for third-party risks is essential and prudence suggests that this should be a joint partnership responsibility. Another insurance which is essential for individual doctors is an insurance with a medical defence organisation. These organisations provide advice and legal defence for any member who is threatened with legal proceedings by a patient. It is usually a precondition of entering a partnership that a general practitioner should be so insured and that this insurance should be kept up to date.

Whether the purchase of books and journals is undertaken by the practice or by individual doctors is also a matter for partnership agreement. In view of the rising cost of books it would seem sensible to pool resources rather than risk duplication.

B. Practice from Health Centres

For those doctors who work in health centres there is a consolidated service charge levied by the District Health Authority (Red Book para. 53.2) and deducted by the FPC from the quarterly payments. This charge covers staff costs, insurance of premises, telephone, heat and light, laundry, repairs and redecorations. It does not cover the employment of staff personally by the general practitioner or the renewal of personal medical equipment.

As the rent charged for the premises by the District Health Authority is reimbursed by the Department of Health and Social Security through the Family Practitioner Committee, this transaction takes place above the head of the general practitioner as a book-keeping transaction from one government pocket to another. The proportion of the health centre rates which are payable by the general practitioner for the rooms his practice uses are similarly directly reimbursed. If the general practitioner in a health centre employs his own staff, he does so under the same terms and conditions as if he were in private accommodation.

The annual service charges are fixed by the District Health Authority. It is usual for the general practitioners using the health centre to pay an agreed percentage of the total cost of running the health centre under each separate heading. For example, they might agree to pay 25 per cent of the wages of the cleaner, 20 per cent of heating and lighting costs, 50 per cent of the telephone rental and 100 per cent for the furniture in their consulting-rooms. The provisional charge for the current year is based on the latest known annual cost of running the centre. As the health centre accounts may be up to two years in arrears, the balancing charge to the general practitioners using the health centre may be considerable in these inflationary times.

If the practitioners think the percentage is unreasonably high, they may discuss the matter with the DHA. If after discussion practitioners are not satisfied with the assessment, they may ask for the matter to be referred to arbitration in accordance with paragraph 10 of the Model Health Centre Licence (Circular HC77/8 Appendix B) which was issued to all Area Health Authorities in April 1977.

Capital Expenses

Capital expenses are non-recurring. They are those which are involved in buying or building something new. Every purchase whether it be furniture, office equipment or medical equipment is technically a capital charge whether it is bought for the first time or is a replacement. Repairs to the practice premises are running expenses; building on an extension or converting a larder into a lavatory are capital expenses. The running costs of a car are a running expense, while the cost of buying a new car (although it may be in replacement of an old one) is a capital expense.

The capital expenses of running a practice depend almost entirely on the philosophy of the partners.

All Expenses

Many practices have in the past been ill-equipped and the standards accepted in waiting rooms, offices and consulting rooms have been lamentably low. It has taken general practitioners a long time to realise that the money which they as a profession spend on their practices as a legitimate expense is reimbursed through the 'expense factor' portion of their remuneration. From sampling a number of practices over a period of ten years it has become clear that in addition to wide variations between practices as to the level of expenses which they incur (examples in Section 2), some practices are still not claiming against tax all the expenses to which they are entitled. A model form of income and expenditure devised by the GMSC for use by general practitioners is shown in Section 2 of this chapter. Practitioners are strongly urged to ensure that their accountants present their returns to the income tax authorities in this way. The wider implications of claims by individual practices are discussed at the end of this chapter, and analyses of income and expenditure as the basis of financial management in a practice in Chapter 19.

Special Points

1. Personally or Practice?

Whether certain expenses should be borne by the practice, or personally by the partners, is a difficult question. It can only be decided by each partnership for itself. In some practices the expense of buying and running one car for each partner is borne by the practice. This has the advantage that if the purchase of a car results in an overdraft, a practice overdraft attracts tax relief whereas a private overdraft does not. On the other hand, in the past many general practitioners had cars that were expensive both to buy and run because 'it was on the practice'.

A similar question arises in the purchase of medical equipment. For equipment or furniture which is more complicated and expensive it is essential that there should be a practice policy both for purchase and disposal. The partnership agreement should cover such matters to prevent misunderstandings and arguments. It is important that the practice accountant should receive from each partner a full list of the expenses he has personally incurred in the course of his professional duties as well as the practice list of shared expenses.

2. *Lease or Buy?*

Whether to rent furniture, equipment or cars, should be considered by partnerships and individual practitioners. The total cost of leasing and renting is allowed against tax as a running expense. If the purchase of an expensive item were to increase a personal overdraft (against the interest on which tax is not allowed) then it might be cheaper to lease than to buy. But no general rules apply, and each case must be worked out using the actual figures involved.

3. *Wife's Salary*

The extent to which a general practitioner's wife takes part in the running of the practice varies enormously from practice to practice, from urban area to rural area. She may be a fully-fledged member of the practice staff, she may have very little connection with the practice except for answering the telephone when her husband is on call (taking and recording messages, making appointments, sometimes reception and nursing duties, answering questions and giving advice). But however little or much she does it should be axiomatic that she is paid the rate for the job. If she is paid more than a certain amount per week (1984 £34.00) both she and her employer become liable for National Insurance contributions. In addition, if she earns more than £38.50 (1984) PAYE is deductible at source. If the practitioner is female the same conditions regarding salary and pension may apply to her husband.

4. *Wife's Pension*

As an employee in the practice the practitioners' wives are entitled to a pension the premiums of which are tax-free. All employing practitioners would be well advised to weigh the merits of the various schemes which are available.

5. *Doctor's Residence*

Many general practitioners see patients at their own homes during the evenings and weekends they are on call. As recognition of the fact that the rooms in the house which may be used by patients have to be furnished, lit, and heated, it is customary for the tax authorities to allow a proportion of the expenses involved in running the doctor's house (rent, rates, repairs, heating, lighting, cleaning, and so on) to be set against income tax. Obviously in some practices this does not apply, but different inspectors may allow 25 per cent to 50 per cent of such costs to be set against income, according to the amount of use a doctor makes of his residence for these purposes. If a practitioner who claims part of the running expenses of his own home against his income tax sells his house at a profit he becomes liable to capital gains tax on that portion he has claimed against tax. If, however, he buys another house from which he is also going to practice in a similar way then the capital gain can be 'rolled over'. If this situation arises a practitioner should seek up-to-date advice from his accountant.

6. Bank Charges

Under the present regulations (1984) when the interest on a practice overdraft is allowed against tax but that on a personal overdraft is not, many young practitioners will find it advantageous to negotiate with their practice bank manager. Payment for all the work we do is in arrears — sometimes up to a year. In these circumstances most bank managers are willing to grant a practice overdraft, the limit depending on the practice net income. It would obviously be foolish to borrow so much that difficulties might arise. It is doubtful whether the bank manager would sanction it in any case. However, a practice overdraft of up to 10 per cent of the net income should not under any circumstances cause any embarrassment and could well be a help to a young practitioner entering practice.

National Insurance Contributions

There are four classes of National Insurance contributions. All general practitioner principals are required to pay Class 2 contributions (i.e. those for the self-employed). Most general practitioners will also be liable to pay Class 4 contributions as well. These are a supplement payable by the self-employed if their income is above a certain level. Some general practitioners, i.e.

those who are employed part-time in other spheres, will also be liable to pay Class 1 contributions as employees. Fortunately, there is an overall limit to the contributions demanded, and practitioners are strongly advised to apply through their accountants for deferment or exemption if they have reasonable grounds for doing so.

National Insurance benefits are only related to the Class 2 contributions (self-employed) even if Class 1 payments are also made. Hence general practitioners working as employed persons (part-time) cannot claim the higher employed person's benefits even though they pay the higher contributions.

Superannuation

For general practitioners 6 per cent of the superannuable earnings received through the FPC are deducted at source. In this context 'superannuable earnings' means the total income received from the FPC minus a figure calculated to represent practice expenses. Contributions cease on retirement. The benefits which a general practitioner may receive under the scheme include:

(1) A lump sum, which is tax-free and payable on retirement

(2) A retirement pension which is payable on retirement at 60 or after. It is paid from the age of 70 whether a general practitioner continues to work or not.

(3) An incapacity allowance and pension to a doctor who after five years' service has to retire owing to ill-health.

If a general practitioner dies in harness his family may receive:

(1) A death gratuity
(2) A widow's pension.
(3) A child's allowance.

The pension which a general practitioner receives depends on the total of his superannuable earnings over his career within the National Health Service. The annual pension is 1.4 per cent (or about 1/70) of his total superannuable earnings. In 1972, in view of inflation, the Board of Inland Revenue agreed that each year's earnings should be 'dynamised'. Each year from 1948 to the present has been allocated a dynamising factor. The dynamising factor for 1960 to 1961 for example is 3.947. This means that in the calculation of total superannuable income, the sum credited to a general practitioner is the sum which he was informed was his superannuable pay in 1960 to 1961 multiplied by 3.947. In this way the pension earned by a general practitioner in his working life is not made obsolete by inflation.

The regulations concerning superannuation are exceedingly complex. If further information is needed the Department of Health and Social Security published a guide to the NHS Superannuation Scheme in 1974 which is available from Her Majesty's Stationery Office. A 'Practitioners' Supplement' to this guide was produced in 1977 and can be obtained from the DHSS Health Services Superannuation Division.

The General Medical Services Committee (further discussed in Chapter 24) negotiate the terms of general practitioners' superannuation and their secretariat can provide up-to-date information on request.

Added Years

Until recently it was possible for practitioners to purchase an additional lump sum for retirement and additional added years on very advantageous terms. These concessions were negotiated by the GMSC to enable older practitioners whose career had started before the beginning of the Health Service to increase their pension rights so that they would be able to retire on a reasonable pension. Now that this generation is passing the regulations have been changed. It is still possible to purchase added years, but the 'premium' is fixed as a percentage of superannuable pay. Should superannuable pay increase so does the premium. In addition once a practitioner is committed the contract is non-cancellable. Practitioners are well advised to look carefully at the scheme and take professional advice before committing themselves.

Staff Pensions

From April 1978 it became obligatory for an employer to offer each full-time employee either participation in the State Pension Scheme or participation in an approved private pension scheme. If prior to this a practitioner had arranged a private pension scheme for his staff then, provided the scheme and staff meet certain strict criteria (52.9), the employer's contributions, called 'qualifying superannuation contributions', are reimbursable in full on application to the FPC. There are two further important aspects to these regulations. Although no staff appointed to new posts are eligible, pension contributions for new staff appointed to take the place of staff who were eligible are reimbursable (52.9e). Secondly, increased contributions to the pension scheme in line with increases in salary are acceptable for reimbursement, provided they meet the criteria.

All contributions by employers to staff pension schemes should be entered as a practice expense for income tax purposes whether reimbursed or not.

Income Tax

By virtue of their independent-contractor status, general practitioners are self-employed. As such they are taxed under Schedule D for all payments received from the Family Practitioner Committee and many, but not all, of their other earnings. Under Schedule D all expenses incurred 'wholly and exclusively for professional purposes' are deducted from gross fees received to determine net taxable income.

Personal allowances, such as children's allowance, allowances for life insurance policies and wife's earned income allowance, are deducted from the net taxable income and income tax levied on the remainder. Thus the calculation for a single-handed general practitioner is simple:

a = income from PFC
b = expenses of practice
c = personal allowances
d = taxable income

$$a - (b + c) = d$$

Complicating factors are:

(1) Income from other sources from which tax has not been deducted (p).

(2) Income from other sources from which tax (t) has been deducted (q).

So the equation becomes: a − (b + c) + p + q = d

But when the tax on d has been determined (T) a certain amount has already been paid (t). So tax due = T − t.

This attempt to simplify matters may have confused some, but we hope it will have underlined how important it is, if a general practitioner has several sources of income, for the accountant to be informed of the exact amount earned from different sources and any tax paid under Schedule E (PAYE) or on tax paid shares, interest, or on building society interest, so that the assessment may be accurate. Any inaccuracies are more likely to be to the advantage of the income tax inspector than the general practitioner!

To make matters even more difficult when general practitioners practise in partnership it is the partnership which owes the tax on partnership income and not the individual practitioners.

The position is then calculated as follows:

Partners A: B: C
Personal allowances Ac Bc Cc
Total income of partnership 1
Total expenses of partnership E
Personal practice expenses Ab Bb Cb
Tax payable by partnership = tax on 1 − E − (Ac + Ab) − (Bc + Bb) − (Cc + Cb).

When the tax payable by the partnership has been determined it is divided between the partners according to their percentage of partnership income, minus (less) their personal allowances and expenses.

For capital expenses involved in building something new or converting part of a building for practice purposes, there is no tax allowance. There is, however, an improvement grant scheme (para 56.1 in the Red Book) which is discussed further in Chapter 11. It cannot be emphasised too strongly that the Family Practitioner Committee must approve the project *before* any contract is signed or work begun otherwise the grant will not be payable.

For the capital expense of buying new furniture or new equipment a capital allowance is made by the income tax authorities. Since 1972 the amount of the purchase price which can be set against tax in the year of purchase is up to 100 per cent at the discretion of the tax payer. If he does not choose to set the whole amount against tax in the first year, then the tax allowance in following years on the remainder is 25 per cent. The one exception to this ruling is the purchase of a car. When a car is purchased only 25 per cent of the price is allowed to be set against tax in the first year as it is in succeeding years.

Example: for a car which costs £4,000, 25 per cent (= £1,000) would be set against tax in the first year, i.e. the purchaser would not have to pay tax on £1,000 of his income. For the next year the 'written down' value of the car would be £3,000 and 25 per cent of this sum (i.e. £750) would be set against tax for that year. For the third year the written down value would be £2,250 and so on. If the car is sold at any time for more than the written down value, the tax authorities can claim back the excess part of the tax relief allowed in previous years. The last proviso applies not only to cars but also to sales of all capital equipment on which allowances have been claimed.

The running expenses of a car, which include not only petrol, oil, servicing, but repairs, licence and insurance, are allowed against tax annually — but a proportion (usually 10 per cent) is agreed with the tax authorities as being for private rather than professional use, and this proportion of the total expense is not allowed.

Wider Implications

This chapter has of necessity been complicated. It has been hard going both to read and to write. Unfortunately, this turgidity reflects the complexity of the systems described — income tax, superannuation, and practice expenses in general.

But the importance of the subject to all general practitioners is undisputed. This is not only for personal reasons but because of the way in which the 'Practice Expense Factor' is calculated. Each year the Review Body, following representations by the BMA and the DHSS, fixes a target net income which they judge right at the time for the average general practitioner with an 'average' list to receive from the National Health Service. To this figure is added a sum to represent practice expenses. The total cake (target net income plus expense factor for all the general practitioners in the country) is then divided into its various slices (capitation fees, basic practice allowance, and so on). See Figure 18.1.

The 'expense factor' which forms the bottom layer of the cake in Figure 18.1 is calculated by taking the tax returns of 15 per cent of the practices in the country, extracting and averaging and legitimate expenses claimed and adding a best guess to make up for inflation since the returns were made. For the year 1984/5 the expense factor was fixed at £10,830 in April 1984. The expense factor is based on expenses actually incurred and declared by practitioners. There are two direct consequences. Firstly, that if *all* general practitioners employed good staff and paid them properly, bought the equipment necessary for their work, and upgraded their premises then these expenses would be reflected in the expense factor within five years and reimbursed to *all* general practitioners. Secondly, that if practitioners do not claim their legitimate

Figure 18.1

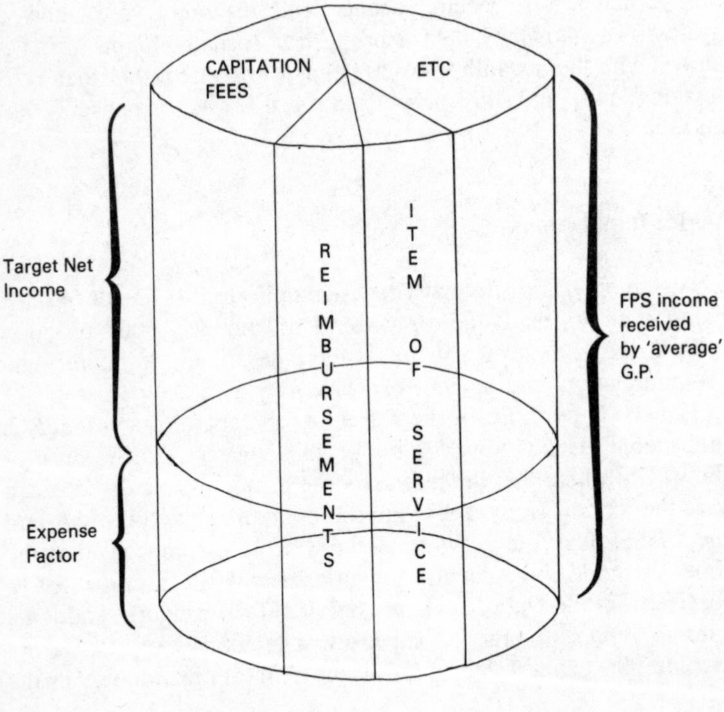

expenses in full against tax then not only will they themselves be paying more tax than they need, but general practice as a whole will suffer by a diminution of the expense factor.

We believe that in spite of advice from accountants and exhortations from many sides, many practices still do not accurately reflect their expenses in the accounts. It is in the interest of the whole profession that they do so.

Further Reading

BMA. *Members' Handbook*, Section V: Superannuation (BMA, 1977).

Practitioners' supplement to the *Guide on National Health Service Superannuation for England and Wales*. DHSS Health Services Superannuation Division (Hesketh House, 200/220 Broadway, Fleetwood, Lancs).

Report of the General Medical Services Committee to the Annual Conference of Representatives of Local Medical Committees 1977. Appendix II: Memorandum on Practice Expenses (BMA, 1977).

Chapter 18: Section 2

A. The following form for recording income and expenditure has been designed by the General Medical Services Committee for the use of general practitioners and their accountants. An aide-mémoire *regarding expenses is attached. Practitioners are urged to ensure that their accountants are aware of this form and use it in presenting their accounts.*

Model form of income and expenditure account for use by general practitioners

Doctors ....

Income and expenditure account for the year ended ....198............

EXPENDITURE

Medical expenses	xx	
Drugs, dressings etc		
Sundry equipment etc	xx	
		xxx
Premises		
Rent (including paid to health centres)	xx	
Rates	xx	
Fuel, light, power and water	xx	
Insurance (building and contents)	xx	
Exterior and interior maintenance and decorations	xx	
Cleaning, etc	xx	
Interest — (building society and other loans in connection with purchase of premises including interest on group practice loans)	xx	
		xxx
Staff costs (wages, national insurance and superannuation contributions)		
Assistants	xx	
Trainees	xx	
Dispensers, receptionists and other staff (including salaries relating to wives)	xx	
Staff advertising and agency fees	xx	
		xxx
Locum and other deputising costs		xxx
Car and travel		
Car rental	xx	
Tax and insurance	xx	
Petrol, oil and repairs	xx	
Taxi and other travel expenses	xx	
		xxx
Other expenses		
Telephone	xx	
Postage	xx	

Stationery, magazines and technical literature	xx	
Professional and other subscriptions	xx	
Refresher courses and professional training	xx	
Medical committee expenses	xx	
Laundry and dry cleaning	xx	
Accountancy and legal	xx	
Bank interest and charges (not related to properties)	xx	
Hire purchase charges	xx	
Superannuation (practitioners)	xx	
Sundry	xx	
		xxx
Depreciation and amortisation		
Premises	xx	
Cars	xx	
Equipment	xx	
		xxx
		xxxx
Net income for the year		xxxx
		£xxxx

INCOME

Family Practitioner Committees		
Fees and other payments for medical services (including dispensing)	xxx	
Reimbursements for:		
Premises (rented and owned including health centres)	xx	
Ancillary help	xx	
Trainees	xx	
Locums	xx	
		xxx
Local authorities and other government departments etc		xxx
Other (including private)		xxx
Income assessed under Schedule E		
Net fees	xx	
P.A.Y.E. deductions	xx	
Superannuation and other deductions	xx	
		xxx

Footnotes:

1. It is important to ensure that payments received from FPCs in respect of part or complete reimbursement of expenses are shown as income and any deductions therefrom by way of health centre expenses, medical committee expenses etc, shown as expenditure.
2. All expenses should include VAT attributable to that expense.
3. If more than one surgery is used it may be informative to show separately the premises expenses relating to each surgery.
4. It may be considered appropriate to make adjustments for private use of motor cars and house expenses in the accounts themselves rather than in the tax computations in which event it would probably be desirable to indicate this fact against the items concerned.

Aide-mémoire — Expenses

Accounting items (heading as in underlined headings of the model form)	Example/comment
1. Medical expenses	
Drugs, dressings and containers	
Disposable equipment and reagents	
Study equipment and replacements not capitalised i.e. not listed under (7)	Auriscope, stethoscope
Repairs and servcing of equipment	ECG machine, typewriter
2. Premises (see Footnote F1)	
A. Privately rented	
Rent	
Rates	General, water, sewage, refuse
Heating, lighting, power	Gas, electricity, oil, solid fuel
Water	If metered
Insurance	Building and contents
Maintenance and decoration	
Cleaning materials/services	
Security alarm system: Rental and maintenance	
B. Premises owned by GPs	
Rent	

Accounting items (heading as in underlined headings of model form)	Example/comment
Practice administrators	
Dispensers	
Receptionists	
Secretaries	
Other practice staff — specify	Physiotherapists etc.
Practitioners' wives	
Cleaners, gardener, car park attendant	
Staff advertising: agency fees	
Uniforms	
Refreshment for ancillary staff	
4. Locum and other deputising costs	
Locum fees	Including agency fees
Aircall (or other deputising services)	
Other locum organisations — specify	
5. Car and travel	
Car rental/hire purchase charges	
Car tax	
Car insurance	
Petrol and oil	

Rates	General, water, sewage, refuse
Heating, lighting, power	Gas, electricity, oil, solid fuel
Water	If metered
Insurance	Building and contents
Maintenance and decoration	
Cleaning materials/services	
Interest	
Mortgage, bank, GP-FC	On premises
Security alarm system: Rental and maintenance	
C. Health centres	
Rent	Notional rent
Rates	General, water, sewage, refuse
Service charge	Building maintenance
Any element in B above not covered by service charge	Telephones
3. Staff costs (see Footnote F1)	
Total gross wages	Before reimbursement from FPC and before deduction of PAYE, Employees' National Insurance and Superannuation contributions

Repairs and maintenance	
Taxi and other travel expenses	
AA/RAC	
Parking and garaging	
6. Other expenses (see Footnote F1)	
Telephones	
Communication equipment	Bleep/radio telephone
Telephone answering service	
Postage	
Printing and stationery	
Magazine and technical literature	Library subscription
Professional subscriptions — specify	GMC, BMA
Subscription to medical defence organization	
Refresher courses and professional training	
Medical committee expenses	Attending AHA, FPC etc.
Laundry and dry cleaning	
Superannuation (practitioners)	
Accountancy, audit, tax and legal fees	
Bank interest charges	Not related to properties
HP charges	Furnishing and equipment
Clothing for doctors	White coats

Aide-mémoire — Expenses

Accounting items (heading as in underlined headings of the model form)	Example/comment	Accounting items (heading as in underlined headings of the model form)	Example/comment
Employers' National Insurance contributions		Levy to LMC	See Footnote F4
Premiums for private pension schemes	Employer's contributions	Other expenses	Periodicals, flowers in waiting room
Sickness and maternity payments		**7. Depreciation and amortisation**	
For: assistants		Cars	
trainees		Equipment, furniture and fittings	
nurses			

Footnotes:

F1. Some groups of doctors have a service company to manage their staff and premises. Such groups should write in for advice to the G.M.S.C. Secretariat at B.M.A. House.

F2 All expenses should include V.A.T.

F3 Each surgery of a multi-storey practice should be itemised separately.

F4 The income from the F.P.C. should be shown as a gross figure on the receipts side before deduction of the contributions to the L.M.C. and an entry of L.M.C. contributions should be shown on the expense side of the accounts.

Source: Sub Appendix B to Appendix II, Report of the General Medical Services Committee to the Annual Conference of Representatives of Local Medical Committees, and the Royal College of General Practitioners Members Reference Book, 1983.

B. Examples of Practice Expenses 1983 in different practices. All amounts are expressed pounds per principal.

	A	B	C	D	E
Staff wages					
Total	16,792	11,950	10,310	18,597	11,570
Reimbursable	9,246	8,978	6,560	13,294	8,440
Non-reimbursable	5,546	2,972	3,750	5,303	3,130
Rent reimbursed	865	2,800	12,450	3,014	3,650
Telephone	525	1,704	1,135	695	1,267
Light and heat	405	332	661	484	564
Postage and printing	77	806	186	347	236
Accounting	859	850	333	603	364
Bank charges	55	1,777	215	120	82
Laundry	—	100	—	267	200

19 BOOK-KEEPING AND ACCOUNTS

For most aspiring partners and many established practitioners, book-keeping is a bore, but whether we like it or not we are in business. The quality and range of services we can offer depends to a considerable extent on the efficiency with which the financial side of our businesses are managed.

The basis of accounting is good book-keeping. It *is* possible to put all the practice bank statements and cheque stubbs in a sack and deliver them to the accountant — but this is a very expensive way of going about things.

The first stage in organisation of practice finance is to keep two cash books, one for cash received and one for expenditure. Both should have analysis columns which can be headed appropriately for the practice. Usually the practice decides on its own headings without reference to the headings the accountant uses in his subsequent analysis. It can save time and expense to confer and agree.

Another deficiency which can give rise to trouble but which can be easily corrected is to ensure that all standing orders and direct debits are entered in the expenditure book, and that credits paid directly into the bank are entered in the income book. Examples of pages of income and expenditure books may be found in Section 2. In this way the analysis books contain a full picture of practice income and expenditure which can be used by the accountant in the preparation of the accounts. The figures also can be used for comparison and discussion within the practice. This aspect is discussed further in Chapter 20.

Profit and Loss Account

Working from the analysis books it is possible to itemize the sources and amount of income and expenditure. The gross income received by the practice over the financial year and the total expenses can be calculated, subtraction of total expenses from the gross income giving the net income or profit.

This calculation is usually carried out by the partnership accountant who will present the profit and loss (i.e. income and

Figure 19.1: Drs A, B and C, Income and Expenditure Account for the year ended 31 December 1982

1981				
		INCOME		
		Family Practitioner Committee		
	81,018	Fees		84,411
		Reimbursement for:		
7,979		Premises	32,679	
—		Doctors Retainer Scheme	1,181	
17,108		Ancillary Help	26,333	
—		Dispensing	1,244	
10,023		Trainees	10,695	
	35,110			72,132
	116,128			156,543
	80	Local Authorities		—
	7,019	University		7,534
	2,588	Other Fees (including Private)		4,899
	—	Taxed Interest Received (Net)		143
	125,815	GROSS INCOME RECEIVED IN YEAR		169,119
	69,090	Less: Expenditure — per schedule attached		99,783
	£56,725	NET INCOME FOR THE YEAR		£69,336
		EXPENDITURE		
		Medical Expenses		
1,639		Drugs, Dressings, etc	1,557	
445		Sundry Equipment	—	
	2,084			1,557
		Premises		
5,847		Rent	2,525	
2,110		Rates	2,433	
1,071		Fuel, Light and Power	1,732	
119		Insurance	596	
2,937		Exterior and Interior maintenance	624	
—		Interest charged on building loan	24,909	
	12,084			32,819
		Staff Costs		
—		Locum	1,845	
10,470		Wages — Trainees	9,848	
20,671		— Other	29,386	
8,920		— Employers NIC	3,469	
4,343		— Pension Contributions	5,325	
—		Doctors Retainer Scheme	976	
	44,404			50,849
		Other Expenses		
2,002		Telephone	3,790	
225		Postage	287	
148		Printing and Stationery	494	
56		Technical Books	10	
300		Subscriptions	312	
1,610		Accountancy and Legal	1,600	
508		Bank Charges	937	
3,858		Superannuation Partners	4,514	
60		LMC Levy	61	
436		Sickness Insurance	436	
982		Sundry	1,386	
333		Depreciation	731	
	10,518			14,558
	£69,090	TOTAL EXPENDITURE		£99,783

expenditure account) as soon after the year end as the sums have been agreed. In the sample shown in Fig 19.1 it will be seen that a comparison is made between the current levels (on the right) and the previous year's figures (on the left). It will also be noted that in these particular accounts a large item for 'interest paid' appears under Premises in the schedule of expenses. During the year in question the practice was in the process of building and moving into new premises. The consequences of this will also appear in the balance sheet (Fig. 19.3).

Partners' Capital Accounts

As part of the balance sheet the practice will also be provided with figures showing the drawings of the partners as against the amount they should have drawn. These latter figures are calculated by applying the rules for division of profit in the practice agreement to the net income for the year as shown in the profit and loss account.

In this instance it will be seen that the drawings have exceeded the profit by £1,357. This figure is made up of £6 underdrawn by Partner A, £129 overdrawn by partner B, and £1,234 overdrawn by partner C (last column but one in Figure 19.2).

Balance Sheet

The balance sheet is an annual account of the overall financial position of the partnership. Although there are minor differences in presentation between one accountant and another, all practice balance sheets should include the following components:

1. Statement of capital assets at the beginning and end of the year.
2. Statement of outstanding credits owed to the practice on the last day of the year.
3. The bank balance in the practice account at the end of the year.
4. Statement of outstanding debts owed to the practice on the last day of the year.
5. The total net assets or liabilities of the practice at the end of the year.

Figure 19.2: Drs A, B and C, Partners' Capital Accounts for the year ended 31 December 1982

1981					
		Dr A			
	(579)	Balance at 1 January 1982		747	
		Net Income for the Year			
4,236		Seniority Payment and			
		Superannuation	6,624		
17,194		⅓ Balance	18,806		
21,430			25,430		
20,104		Drawings	25,424		
	1,326			6	
	747	Balance at 31 December 1982			753
		Dr B			
	(886)	Balance at 1 January 1982		469	
		Net Income for the Year			
		Seniority Payment and			
2,119		Superannuation	3,783		
17,194		⅓ Balance	18,806		
19,313			22,589		
17,958		Drawings	22,718		
	1,355			(129)	
	469	Balance at 31 December 1982			340
		Dr C			
	(690)	Balance at 1 January 1982		32	
		Net Income for the Year			
		Vocational Training and			
1,244		Superannuation	2,512		
14,738		⅓ Balance	18,805		
15,982			21,317		
15,260		Drawings	22,551		
	722			(1,234)	
	32	Balance at 31 December 1982			(1,202)
	£1,248	TOTAL CAPITAL ACCOUNTS			£(109)

In order to clarify these points a sample balance sheet for the same practice is shown (Fig. 19.3), and the figures are discussed under the headings as in 1 to 5 above.

Capital Assets (Fixed Assets)

These are shown on the balance sheet as two items. Surgical and Office equipment at Cost of Value, introduced (line 1) includes the total value of the equipment owned by the practice, e.g. carpets, curtains, desks, chairs, filing cabinets, medical equipment.

Figure 19.3: Drs A, B and C, Balance Sheet at 31 December 1982

	1981					
			FIXED ASSETS			
(1)		4,280	Surgical and Office Equipment at Cost or Value Introduced			7,256
(2)		2,388	Less: Depreciation to Date			3,119
(3)		1,892				4,137
(4)		131,679	Land and Buildings — at cost			221,521
(5)		133,571				225,658
			CURRENT ASSETS			
(6)	3,018		Debtors and Prepayments		3,790	
(7)	—		Building Society Deposit		11,645	
(8)	35		Cash in Hand		35	
(9)	3,053				15,470	
			LESS: CURRENT LIABILITIES			
(10)	1,050		Creditors and Accrued Expenses	4,389		
(11)	131,679		Bank Loan Account	234,700		
(12)	2,647		Bank Overdraft	2,148		
(13)	135,476				241,237	
(14)		(132,323)	NET CURRENT LIABILITIES			(225,767)
(15)		£1,248	NET ASSETS/(LIABILITIES)			£(109)
(16)		£1,248	FINANCED BY PARTNERS CAPITAL ACCOUNTS			£(109)

We have prepared, without carrying out an audit, the above Balance Sheet at 31 December 1982 and annexed Income and Expenditure Account for the year ended on that date from the accounting records of our clients and from information and explanations supplied to us.

Snooks, Bloggs & Co.
Chartered Accountants
Mole House
The Wood
Exeter

At the beginning of 1982 the figure in the sample balance sheet was £7,256. The comparable figure for 1981 was £4,280 from which it can be deduced that £2,976 of capital equipment was bought during the year. The figure of £3,119 (line 2) is the cumulative depreciation which has occurred since the assets were acquired, so that the figure of £4,137 (line 3) is the total written down value of the fixed assets owned by the practice, apart from land and buildings, at the end of 1982. The balance sheet shows that the value of land and buildings owned by the partnership grew from £131,679 to £221,521 (line 4) in the course of 1982. The total value of fixed assets on 31 December 1982 is shown as £225,658 (line 5).

Outstanding Credits

These are listed under the heading Current Assets. They include items which are due to the practice for work carried out during the year 1982 for which payment is expected after the year end, i.e. in 1983 (debtors). It also includes estimates for payments which have been made in 1982 in advance for such items as rent, insurance and rates occurring in 1983 (prepayments, line 6). These figures are difficult to estimate because many items of NHS practice income are paid in arrears. It is usual, therefore, to include receipt for many such items during the year they are received rather than in the year they were earned. This does not matter from the point of view of comparing practice accounts from one year to another provided that a consistent policy is followed. However, if such payments are included one year in the 'year earned' and in another in 'year received' this can produce considerable distortion in apparent profits. Any building society deposits (line 7) or cash in hand (line 8) are also included under current assets.

The Bank Balance

The balance on the last day of the year is entered under current assets if in credit, or under current liabilities (line 12) if there is an overdraft.

Outstanding Debts (Current Liabilities)

These are debts incurred by the practice but unpaid on the day the books closed. In the sample the figure of £4,389 quoted for 'creditors and accrued expenses' (line 10) is composed of items such as PAYE for staff (incurred but not paid), bills for professional services (e.g. to accountants) which are presented in arrears, estimated outstanding accounts for telephones and electricity.

Total Net Assets and Liabilities

In order to obtain the total net liabilities of the practice at the end of the financial year the current assets (line 9) are subtracted from the current liabilities (line 13). Subtraction of this figure, i.e. £225,767 (line 14), from the fixed assets (line 5) gives the total net assets/liabilities of the practice at the year end as minus £109 (line 16).

Interpretation of Accounts

When a practitioner, whether trainee aspiring partner or established principal, is looking at the accounts of a practice it is easy to be mazed by figures. It may be difficult to translate the figures on the page into aspects of life in the practice. The following guidance may be useful.

1. The level of gross income and the sources from which it comes can be found in the income and expenditure account. Examination of these figures will show what proportion of the practice activities is concerned with the Health Service and how much work the practice undertakes outside the NHS. It will also show the scale of reimbursements obtained on premises and staff salaries.

2. The level of expenditure incurred in running the practice and the proportion spent on individual items can also be ascertained from the income and expenditure account. The practice philosophy towards premises, towards remuneration of staff, and towards purchase of medical books, for example, will show itself by the proportion of expenditure incurred under these headings.

3. The philosophy of the practice towards expenditure can be further substantiated by looking at the change in the value of fixed assets on the balance sheet. Comparison of the figures for the current year and the previous year will reveal the capital expenditure on new equipment/furnishings undertaken by the practice during the financial year.

4. The overall level of fixed assets shown on the balance sheet, giving an indication of the equipment, furniture and property owned by the practice, will have considerable financial significance for doctors joining and leaving the practice.

5. Examination of the partners' capital accounts will throw light on the partnership agreement concerning division of profits. Enquiry will reveal the relationship between division of profit and division of work, including possibly retention of fees for certain categories of work. Many other aspects of internal partnership organisation may come to light when these figures are considered.

6. Income tax paid by the partnership. In some practice accounts information concerning tax liabilities may be found either under 'current liabilities' or as an item reserving money against future tax changes. Comparison of the tax paid with the level of total practice expenditure can provide insight into the way the

practice views the relationship between expenditure on patients and contributions to the tax authorities.

Summary

The ability to understand and to draw inferences about the running of a practice from the annual accounts is essential for young doctors who are applying for practice vacancies. In the interests of good financial management, we believe it is equally important that established principals should be able to interpret the accounts of their own practices.

Chapter 19: Section 2

Examples of pages from the financial analysis books of a three-partner practice

(a) Income

Date	Source	Amount of cheque or cash	Paid to bank	Insur. Company	Medical Reports	Crema-tions	Private Patients	Health Authority	NHC Dental Anaesthetics Retainer Scheme	Direct Credits	Sundries
1982	Brought Forward	102471.20	102471.20	793.50	294.90	207.00	441.00	945.28	468.64	9619.46	2875.42
Sept 29	Dept of Transport										
	(H. Sinclair)	5.30			5.30						
	University of Exeter	509.61	509.61							509.61	
	Luxton (re Jock Deed)	15.50				15.50					
	Telecom refund (JM 21644)	18.14									
Oct 6	Timkin Jun Qtr	21.00					21.00				
	etc.			etc.							
Oct 13	NCH Qtr ended 30.9.82	71.38							71.38		
Oct 20	Norwich Un. Ins.										
	(D. Weston)	8.25		8.25							
	Prudential Ass. (I. Sprocket)	18.00		18.00							
	DHA (Bed fun)	20.60						20.60			
	Carried Forward	121764.31	121653.37	974.25	327.05	238.00	465.00	1000.57	540.02	115070.30	2879.62

(b) Expenditure

Date	Paid to	Amount of cheque	Salaries /Wages	Profess. Charges, Income tax	Rates /Rent	Insurance, Postage	Electric, Phone	R & R Maint. Furniture	Office Equipm. Surgical print & Stat.	Direct Debits Standing Orders	Petty Cash, Sundries
1982	Brought forward	126273.08	42341.96	22067.03	2983.24	748.50	4156.94	2731.70	1798.34	48247.30	1198.07
Nov 1	Dr P.H.W. Locum × 6	90.00	90.00								
	Dr G.M. (6 sessions)	120.00	120.00								
Nov 2	Scottish Amicable	205.07								205.07	
	Petty cash	64.30	55.20			4.65					4.45
	SW Water Authority	296.89			296.89						
	etc.				etc.						
17	Harbour printing	29.12							29.12		
	SW Electr. Board	12.60					12.60				
	Petty Cash	59.12	18.40			16.80			2.75		21.18
24	Inland Rev.M7 (PAYE 546.60, NI 508.88)	1055.48		1055.48							
	Carried forward	132212.64	44840.93	23122.51	3280.13	807.45	4169.54	2731.70	2052.12	49948.06	1260.20

20 FINANCIAL MANAGEMENT

Before discussing ways in which the financial activities of a practice may be managed it is necessary first to define what these activities are.

Basic Financial Operations

Certain operations are undertaken by all (or almost all) practices. They can be summarised as follows:

Income

1. Receive note and bank all in-coming items.
2. Send off claims for reimbursement (e.g. staff salaries, employers share of NI, staff pensions, doctors retainer scheme) together with receipts for rents, general rates and water rates. Check amounts which are reimbursed.
3. Make out bills (e.g. for private patients): send out: cross check when received
4. Check outstanding accounts.
5. Send claim for trainee to FPC mid-month if applicable.

Expenditure

1. Pay accounts as and when due after checking accuracy: obtain receipts.
2. Pay salaries of staff (after obtaining overtime list) obtain receipt for salaries paid from petty cash.
3. Do PAYE and NI table. Fill amounts to be paid in the book supplied by the Inland Revenue. Send off cheque for total amounts due by 19th of each month.
4. Purchase NI stamp for doctors. Stamp up card. Obtain new card annually.
5. Maintain petty cash float.

Bank Statements

1. Check that amounts are correct.
2. Check standing orders and direct debits.

3. Make sure all entries on the statement belong to the practice.

Changes

Under this heading are grouped changes in the practice which have direct financial implications.

1. *In Staff*
   a. Note changes in staff or hours worked, submit revised ANCI to FPC. Record all details on salary record and pay record forms.
   b. For staff leaving: prepare and deal with Form P45: send Part I to the Inland Revenue.
   c. For incoming staff: obtain P45 and NI card (only when exempt or at reduced rate), fill in Part 2 of P45 and send to Inland Revenue, retain Part 3.
   d. For staff away on sick leave: fulfil statutory sick pay regulations.
   e. For staff pensions: if linked to salaries when salaries are changed advise the insurance company to prepare new policies. If appropriate forward new policy to FPC for revised reimbursement.
2. *In premises*
   a. Note any changes in rates, rents, lease. Submit revised PREM form to FPC retaining a copy.
   b. Note future dates for reassessments which affect reimbursements.

Extended Financial Operations

The above list contains jobs which have to be done in all practices which employ staff, use premises, and undergo changes. They comprise the inescapable foundation for running the financial side of an efficient general practice. The next step is to organise the book-keeping and records using simple income and expenditure analysis as described in Chapter 19. When this information is accurate and regularly available further analyses can be made.

1. **Extended income analysis:** the column headings in the income book may be sufficient for tax and general accounting purposes, but in order to obtain a more detailed picture of practice activity it is necessary to set out items of income in a way which

reflect all sources of income. One method we ourselves use is to list all NHS fees and allowances received under the headings contained in the quarterly account which is received from the FPC. To this are added headings for reimbursements, other NHS income and non NHS income. The totals are cross-checked. The result is a detailed analysis of the sources of practice income and their relative importance for one year. This exercise can be repeated year on year.

2. **Extended expenditure analysis:** a similar exercise can be carried out using more detailed headings for expenditure.

As a result of such analysis a practice can possess a consistent and comparable picture of its financial performance related to its activities over a number of years. An example of the way a four-year comparison in a three-partner practice can be set out is given in Section 2 of this chapter.

Who Should Manage?

It is only over the past fifteen years or so that the financial side of general practice has become so complex. Prior to PAYE, staff pensions, reimbursements, increased number of staff employed, and complicated national insurance regulations, life was relatively simple. It was commonplace for the senior partner to undertake responsibility for 'the books' with occasional help from a part-time secretary. We know this situation still exists in some practices. We suggest that partners should seriously consider whether this is the most productive way for a doctor to spend his/her time. The arithmatic is irrefutable. For an hour in which he carries out two insurance medicals a practitioner can earn £34.00 (1984). In the same hour a senior secretary or finance secretary doing the books will be paid say £3.00 (1984) of which £2.10 will be reimbursed; net cost 90p. The cost of an accountant's clerk carrying out the same operation on behalf of the practice will be of the order of £25.00 per hour (1984). This is not to say we recommend that all responsibility for financial affairs should be abrogated by the partners, only that they should seriously look at those aspects of day-to-day book-keeping (such as form filling and analysis) which can equally well be undertaken by someone other than themselves. It is our experience that a good secretary or finance secretary can relieve practitioners of humdrum book work, can provide (and enjoy providing) figures using which doctors can exercise their management responsibilities, and can reduce the amount of money paid to accountants for routine checking by their clerks. The role of a practice accountant under this scenario is changing. General practitioners have in the past tended to view their accountants as someone who sorted out their figures in order to plead their cause to the tax inspector. With the advent of basic book-keeping within practices and increasing knowledge among practitioners of the issues involved it is possible for accountants to move into the more sophisticated role of financial advisors to the practice, a role for which their training and expertise has prepared them.

Why Bother?

Many practitioners may find the ideas expressed above distasteful and will query the need to alter established routine. They will question whether the time and effort put into carrying out analysis is worthwhile. The arguments for such involvement can be listed as follows:

1. Reduction of expense: as explained above, employment of a secretary to carry out routine book-keeping costs a practice about 90p an hour after reimbursement and this expense is itself allowed against tax. It would be difficult to find a more inexpensive way of obtaining equivalent services from partners or accountants. Practices which carry out their own initial analysis in co-operation with their accountants have found this fact reflected in the fees they pay.
2. Professional satisfaction: morale within a practice is higher when the partners feel in command of a situation rather than when they feel buffeted by forces they cannot control. This is another aspect of 'audit' discussed in Chapter 15.
3. Attitude of partners: morale is also heightened if partners trust each other, feeling that the relation between workload and profit is open and fair. Analysis and discussion of practice finance is a very potent factor in maintaining such trust.
4. Correction of overspending or underclaiming can be undertaken. A review of, for example, heating or telephone costs can show variations which are not explicable in terms of inflation. A review of income from cervical cytology may reveal that claim forms are not being properly or appropriately filled in.

5. Planning activities: if by analysis the practice can establish trends, or can forecast the position for some time ahead, then forward planning becomes a real possibility. The time to buy equipment or books, the best time to redecorate or improve premises, can be part of a general planning exercise in which the accountant can play an important part.

6. Comparison with other practices: this can be a very illuminating exercise. For example in 1982 the comparable figures for two practices (both non-dispensing) were as shown in Table 20.1.

Table 20.1: Comparison of 1982 Income and Expenditure from Two Similar Practices

	Income and expenditure in £000	
	A: 3 partners	B: 4 partners
FPC income	85	114
Reimbursements	69	22
Non-NHS income	11	26
Total income	167	162
Total expenses	99	44
Available to partners	68	118
Income tax paid	7	48
Drawings by partners	61	70

Translated into terms of per patient per partner the figures emerge as shown in Table 20.2.

Table 20.2: Expenses and Income Expressed Per Patient and Per Partner

	A	B
Gross income per partner	56,000	40,500
Gross income per patient	£29.8	£19
Expenses per partner	33,000	11,000
Expenses per patient	£17.7	£5.1
'Profit' per partner	20,330	17,500
'Profit' per patient	£10.9	£8.2

It is quite clear that practice B spends much less on reimbursable items (premises and staff) and less on other items in the practice, has almost double the income available to partners — and pays nearly seven times as much income tax. It would seem highly likely to say the least that the partners and patients in practice B would benefit from a more detailed financial analysis of the practice income and expenditure.

Summary

Basic and extended financial operations within a practice have been described. The case has been put for undertaking some financial analysis in the practice as an aid to management. There is no doubt that attitudes are changing and that more practitioners now appreciate the direct relationship between financial management and the ability to provide service to patients, staff and partners.

Chapter 20: Section 2

A. *Example of a job description list for a Finance Secretary*

As needed

1. Cheques and payments in — enter in cash ledger and paying in book: bank. Check all outstanding accounts are paid — if not, follow up!
2. Pay accounts as and when due. Get accounts receipted. All local accounts to be delivered. Check that all accounts are technically correct. Take care not to pay for items you haven't had.
3. All debits paid by the practice (name, cheque, number, amount) must be entered in the expenditure analysis book.
4. All income received by the practice must be entered in the income analysis book.
5. Order stationery.
6. Sort SFA amendments and make sure all copies of the Red Book are up to date.
7. Submit ANC 1 for any ancillary staff changes (i.e. hours, rates of pay, new staff, staff leaving). Also record all details of changes on staff salary record and pay record forms.
8. For staff who are leaving prepare and deal with P45. Forward Part 1 to the Inland Revenue and give Parts 2 and 3 to the person leaving.
9. For new staff — obtain P45 and NI card (if exempt from paying NI or if reduced rates are paid). Fill in part 2 of P45 and send to Inland Revenue. Retain Part 3.
10. For changes in the premises fill in a PREM form. Submit in duplicate to the FPC. Retain a copy.
11. Complete statistics and enquiry forms as necessary.
12. Amend standing orders and direct debits at bank as and when necessary.

Weekly

13. Check, write up and replenish petty cash as neccessary. Do analysis for transfer to expenditure book.
14. Do filing.

Monthly

15. Bank statements: check accounts are correct.
16. Balance the bank statements.
17. Cross-check bank statements against entries in the analysis books.
18. Check all standing orders and make sure that all entries on the bank statements belong to the practice.
19. Obtain overtime list for salaries.
20. Work out salaries and make out cheques. If any staff are paid out of petty cash obtain a receipt.
21. Do PAYE and NI table; fill amounts in book (supplied by Inland Revenue); send off cheque for total amount due. This has to be sent by the 19th of each month.
22. Send off claim form to FPC for trainee mid-month: diarise to check reimbursement.

Quarterly

23. Purchase NI stamps for doctors and stamp up card.
24. Private patients: go through appointment sheets for consultations. Check with doctors for visits. Enter amounts in ledger and balance. Make out bills and send out. Cross-check credits against ledger when received.
25. Send off claim forms for reimbursement:

    a. ancillary staff salaries 70% — with separate lists for overtime
    b. staff pensions
    c. doctors' retainer scheme
    d. for the expenses incurred on the premises by health visitors and attached nurses
    e. general rates and water rates
    f. rents: send all receipts
    g. employer's share of employee's NI

    When reimbursement is received check to make sure it is correct.

Annually

26. Total books and analysis columns. Do analysis with breakdown of everything that goes through the account. Prepare books for the accountant.
27. Update doctors' wives' payments and pensions as agreed.
28. Update staff salaries as agreed.
29. Advise company who prepares the policies for staff pensions of the new salaries: forward new documents to FPC in order to receive full reimbursement.
30. Check all practice insurances to ensure that cover is adequate.

End of financial year

31. Go through pay records: total them.
32. Total PAYE and NI: balance. Prepare and send appropriate forms to Inland Revenue.
33. Apply for partners' advance leave payments for new financial year.

B. *Example of an FPC-quarterly advice form issued by Devon FPC — which can be used as a basis for financial analysis*

FAMILY PRACTITIONER COMMITTEE

C. CLARK
Administrator

Dr(s) ______________________________

REMUNERATION OF GENERAL MEDICAL PRACTITIONERS — QUARTER ENDED —

Statement of remuneration payable in accordance with Regulation 24 of the National Health Service (General Medical and Pharmaceutical Services) Regulations 1974.

Total patients on list over 75 years ________ Temporary Residents ________

over 65 years ________ Rural Practice Units ________

under 65 years ________ Dispensing Patients ________

	£	p
1. Basic Practice Allowance		
2. Addition for Group Practice		
3. Addition for Assistant		
4. Capitation Fees: Patients over 75		
5. Patients over 65		
6. Patients under 65		
7. Supplementary Practice Allowance		
8. Supplementary Capitation Fees		
9. Night Visit Fees		
10. Vaccination Fees		
11. Vaccination Fees (Computer)		
12. Cervical Cytology Tests		
13. Maternity Medical Services		
14. Contraceptive Services		
15. Temporary Resident Fees		
16. Emergency Treatment		
17. Anaesthetic Claims		
18. Arrest Dental Haemorrhage		
19. Rural Practice Payments		
20. Dispensing Capitation Fees		
21. Addition for Vocational Training		
22. Addition for Seniority		
23.		
24.		
25.		
26.		

27. R.M.O. Report Fees

GROSS AMOUNT DUE

LESS: DEDUCTIONS

28. Superannuation Contributions (Principals)
29. Superannuation Contributions (Assistants)
30. Advances on Account
31. Health Centre Accounts
32. Leave Payment Recoveries
33. Local Medical Committee Statutory Levy
34. Voluntary Levy
35. Added Superannuation Benefit Contributions
36.
37.
38.

TOTAL DEDUCTIONS

CREDIT TO BANK ON AMOUNT PAYABLE

PLEASE RETAIN THIS STATEMENT FOR YOUR ACCOUNTANT

C: Example of method of presentation of a four-year comparison of income and expenditure

INCOME

	1981	1982	1983	1984
Capitation Temporary residents Contraceptive TOTAL HEAD COUNTS				
Practice Allowances				
Maternity Immunisation Cervical cytology Night visits Emergency treatment TOTAL ITEM OF SERVICE				
Seniority Vocational Training Allowance GP trainer allowance TOTAL PERSONAL				

	1981	1982	1983	1984
Rural practice Group practice Dispensing TOTAL TYPE AND POSITION				
SUNDRIES				
TOTAL FPC PAYMENTS				
Cost rent Rents Rates Wages Pension premiums NI Trainees' salary/allowance Doctors' retainer scheme Nurses and HV Drugs and appliances (see 'dispensing;) TOTAL REIMBURSEMENTS				
TOTAL HOSPITAL PRACTICE				
Insurance medicals National Children's Homes Medical reports Private patients Balance of analysis book Dental anaesthetics University TOTAL NON-NHS PRACTICE				
Standing Order Reversals				
TOTAL INCOME				

RUNNING EXPENSES

Wages: Receptionist Secretary Nursing Cleaning Out of hours: Wives Others Medical locum Doctors' retainer scheme Trainee TOTAL WAGES				

	1981	1982	1983	1984
Employers NI				
Pension:				
Ancillary staff				
Partners' wives				
TOTAL OTHER STAFF COSTS				
TOTAL STAFF COSTS				
Rents: Seaton (M.T.)				
Beer (L.H.)				
Tyr-nan-og				
Branscombe				
For trainee				
Loan account (T.H.)				
TOTAL RENTS				
Rates: General				
Water				
TOTAL RATES				
Repairs/ redecoration				
Insurance				
TOTAL COST OF PREMISES				
Telephone				
Heat and light				
Postage				
Printing and stationery				
TOTAL SERVICING COSTS				
Accounting				
Professional charges				
Bank charges				
Subscriptions				
Journals and books				
Medical drugs/dressings				
Replacement equipment				
Partners' superannuation				
Trainees' superannuation				
Insurances				
LMC levy				
TOTAL PROFESSIONAL COSTS				
General				
Miscellaneous				
Domestic				
TOTAL SUNDRIES				
TOTAL RUNNING COSTS				

CAPITAL COSTS

	1981	1982	1983	1984
Furnishing Office equipment Medical equipment TOTAL PRACTICE CAPITAL COSTS				
TOTAL EXPENDITURE				

SUMMARY

	1981	1982	1983	1984
Standing order reversals				
FPC income Reimbursements Non-NHS income TOTAL income TOTAL expenses				
Partners' standing orders Available to partners Income tax paid Drawings by partners				

PART SIX:

ORGANISATION

21 ROUTINES: YOUR DAY, WEEK AND YEAR

It is no good having a highly organised practice if you yourself are completely disorganised. In fact the two are probably incompatible.

One often reads in the popular press about Dr Bloggs — a busy general practitioner, etc., etc. Busy often equals disorganised, as we can all appear as busy as we wish. This adjective 'busy' frequently appears to be a smoke screen produced by general practitioners to protect them from the demands of the public.

Over the past ten years or so one of the more obvious ways in which doctors have begun to organise themselves is reflected in the fall in home visiting and the decrease in surgeries held after 6 p.m. However, the management of time extends far beyond the manipulation of an appointment system.

Daily Routine

How the partners operate their surgeries depends on many factors, particularly the availability of consulting rooms, patient demand, and other fixed commitments, such as clinical-assistant sessions.

Far too many doctors are fixed in the 9-10.30 a.m. and 5-7 p.m. surgery routine. If each partner has his own consulting room then flexible timetables are possible. However, if consulting rooms have to be shared then some thought will have to be given to the best way to organise this.

It is not a bad idea to have at least one partner consulting on the premises throughout most of the day. In this way a doctor is always on hand to deal with any crisis. This is a valuable back-up facility appreciated by his reception staff. Sessions during the course of the day can also be used for special clinics, such as antenatal, family planning, or geriatric screening clinics.

If one consulting room is being used by two doctors, half-an-hour of 'dead time' between one surgery ending and the next beginning should always be allowed. Almost inevitably the first surgery will not be running exactly to time and there is no reason to stress the doctor further by the knowledge that he has to be out of the room promptly because it is needed by his partner.

Reception staff appreciate clear written instructions which state:

(a) The partners' daily and weekly timetable.
(b) The length of time of each surgery.
(c) The rate of booking required, e.g. eight patients per hour.
(d) The times when insurance medicals and similar items are to be booked, so that these can be arranged without constant referral back to the doctor.
(e) Instructions about receiving and accepting requests for visits. The procedure varies in different practices. It may be that the senior receptionist always deals with these requests or the doctor himself may wish to take the calls. The arrangement should be quite clear and the receptionist should know the details which she should obtain with each message.
(f) The on-call rota of doctors and ancillary staff.

On-call Rota

As the general practitioner's terms of service state that he is responsible for providing medical service for his patients seven days a week, it means that arrangements have to be made for someone always to be available for emergency calls.

A common arrangement is for all partners to take their own calls up until the end of morning surgery, and then for one partner to be available for emergency calls until the end of the evening surgery when the duty doctor for the night takes over.

Whatever rota is decided upon it is important that this is written down so that there is no argument as to who is responsible for taking a late call, and the receptionist should be informed of the whereabouts of the duty doctor throughout the day.

Meetings with Partners and Staff

It is wise to have a fixed time each day or week when the various members of the practice team meet. For instance, it is probably a good idea for the district nurse to see each partner daily to discuss new cases, as well as the changing requirements of patients under their shared care. In a health centre, or premises where she has her own room, this communication is, of course, much easier.

The health visitor and social worker should see each doctor at a fixed time at least once a week to catch up on the various cases. There do not have to be lengthy discussions but these meetings enable everyone to keep in touch with what is happening and certainly prevent any one member of the team from feeling isolated.

Ideally partners should meet each morning over coffee for discussion. However, varying commitments and timetables often mean that one doctor has finished his surgery and is anxious to get away, while another is still consulting, so these meetings do not always occur. In a small practice the partners normally see each other frequently enough to avoid any breakdown in communication, but some thought should be given to this in larger practices. As mentioned elsewhere a regular partnership meeting at least once a month should be arranged in addition to these more informal sessions.

It is particularly important that if one partner is about to take on an extra responsibility, be it a clinical-assistant session or chairmanship of the District Management Team, this matter is discussed fully and freely between the partners before any decision is taken. If the work takes place during practice hours then any income from the work should go into the partnership account and in this way friction is avoided. When the extra commitments are not producing any income, for example, serving on the LMC, then all partners should agree to the arrangement.

When all partners can either share an extra commitment, for example, teaching trainees, or each have a special interest of their own, it is an even better way of avoiding some members of the practice feeling that they are being 'put upon'.

Trainee Responsibility

If a trainee works in the practice then he too should have a written timetable which includes a statement of his teaching sessions with his trainer. Again the reception staff should know how he is to have his patients booked, and what arrangements have been made for his being on call and off duty. Section 2 of this chapter contains the instructions which are given to trainees when they join one of the authors' practices.

The Week

When all these facts are taken into account, the whole of the working week should be clearly structured. The receptionists should have their own instructions as to when to book surgeries, who is on call at any time, and should have no doubt about the procedure they should follow.

The Year

The main planning for the year involves the arrangement for partners and staff holidays. In a theoretical three-partner practice not more than one partner should be on holiday at a time and probably some, if not all, of the partners will want time off during school holidays. If each partner is to have six weeks' holiday, which is fairly average now, then eighteen weeks of the year will see the practice working with two partners only. This means that a different, amended, timetable has to be produced for holiday periods or else a locum is employed to take the place of each partner in the timetable in turn.

Many drug firms now produce large wall charts showing a whole year at a time, and these are very useful for this type of planning. If different colours are used for each partner then these can be marked on the chart for the holiday periods to avoid overlap. Staff holidays can be incorporated on the same chart using different colour codes. It is important that the partners agree in advance who is to have first choice of dates for the year, and that all are agreed on the various holiday entitlements, study leave and sabbatical leave.

It is not intended that this chapter should imply that each doctor must have a rigid timetable to be strictly adhered to at all times irrespective of other considerations. Each doctor must consider his own priorities and incorporate them into his week accordingly. However, with an increasing number of doctors working with more partners and staff it is important that all concerned with the practice are aware of their responsibilities and are also aware of what other members of the practice are doing each day. Only in this way will confusion and arguments be avoided.

We are aware that much of the advice in this chapter is a repetition of advice given elsewhere. This is inevitable. The practice timetable whether over a short or long period reflects the way the practice is organised and the principles of management which form the subject of this book.

Chapter 21: Section 2

A. A typical weekly timetable for a three-partner practice with only two consulting rooms

	9-10.30 a.m.	11-1 p.m.	2-3.30 p.m.	4-6 p.m.	Evening/ Night Duty
Mon	Dr A Dr B Surgery Dr C — Clinical-assistant session	Dr A Dr B Visits	Dr A — Ante-natal clinic Dr B — Insurance medicals	Dr B & Dr C — Surgery ance medicals	
Tues	Dr B — Visits Dr A Dr C Surgery	Dr B — Surgery Dr A Dr C Visits	Dr A — Half-day Dr C — Ante-natal clinic, well woman clinic, FPA session	Dr B — Surgery	Dr C
Wed	Dr A Dr B Surgery Dr C — Visits	Dr A Dr B Visits Dr C — Surgery	Dr B — Half-day	Dr A & Dr C — Surgery	Dr A
Thurs	Dr A — Anaesthetic session Dr B Dr C Surgery	Dr B Dr C Visits	Dr B — Ante-natal clinic Dr C — Half-day	Dr A & Dr B — Surgery	Dr B
Fri	Dr A Dr C Surgery Dr B — Insurance medicals	Dr A Meeting Dr B with Dr C Practice Team & visits	Dr B — Surgery	Dr A & Dr C — Surgery	
Sat	Drs A, B and C in rotation				

Monday: Dr A on call from 11 a.m. to 2 p.m. Dr C on call from 2 to 6 p.m.
Tuesday: Dr C on call from 11 a.m. to 3 p.m. Dr B on call from 3 to 6 p.m.
Wednesday: Dr A on call 11 a.m. to 6 p.m.
Thursday: Dr B on call 11 a.m. to 6 p.m.
Friday: Dr C on call 11 a.m. to 6 p.m.
Each doctor in rotation does 1 in 3 Monday and Friday evening and Saturday/Sunday duty.

B. *Example of a trainee timetable*

The whole essence of any timetable is that it should structure the time available to incorporate all the required activities. It should also be flexible to allow for the changing needs of the persons involved.

The following is a proposed, but negotiable, timetable and it will certainly change from time to time.

	9-11 a.m.	11-1 p.m.	2-4 p.m.	4-6 p.m.
Monday	Surgery	Discussion and visits	Project time and miscellaneous activities	Surgery
Tuesday	Surgery	Visits or morning teaching session in Department	Half-day release course	Surgery
Wednesday	Surgery jointly with trainer	Visits and discussion	2-30-3.30 p.m. Teaching session	Surgery
Thursday	Surgery	Visits	Half-day	
Friday	Surgery	ANC with trainer	Visits 3-3.30 p.m. Teaching session	Surgery

Surgery appointments will be booked at a rate to be decided between the trainee and trainer. In the first six months of the GP year no pressure should be exerted on the trainee's appointment times at all. Visits will be arranged depending on appropriateness, follow-up situation, and practice demand.

Monday afternoon until evening surgery will be used for working on any arranged project or generally catching up on activities. The Wednesday morning surgery is a shared one in which either the trainee or trainer may do the consulting with the other sitting in.

C. Example of information concerning out-of-hours duties for a trainee

---

The philosophy is that the trainee should do the same out-of-hours duties as his trainer. He will, therefore, have a half-day on a Thursday, but this may be changed from time to time if another partner is on holiday. He will do no surgeries or out-of-hours cover without a partner being available for advice and support if necessary.

The evening on duty extends from 6 p.m. to 8.30 a.m. and will normally be alternate Wednesdays with the trainer who will be covering the trainee on his duty night.

The weekend duty includes Friday evening, Saturday morning surgery and then on call until 8.30 a.m. on Monday. It will occur approximately twice in every three months, but will be specified, as different partners in turn will be covering this. At no time is the trainee actually built into the rota; he replaces one partner at a time in turn.

The trainee will also do an occasional Saturday morning surgery and visits when another practitioner is on duty for the weekend.

A separate list of duty dates is enclosed. If a date is inconvenient then there is no objection to the trainee arranging to 'swop' within the rota, provided that the trainer is agreeable.

In the university vacation when there is no half-day release, the trainee will normally do a surgery from 4-5 p.m.

He will also take late and emergency calls which arise after the end of morning surgery on Friday until after the evening surgery when the duty doctor for the weekend takes over.

As already mentioned, the above details are subject to variation in certain circumstances, particularly when one partner is on holiday. The main effect of this would be occasionally moving the half-day to a different day and having to do a night of duty rather than alternate Wednesdays.

---

22 SYSTEMS

One of the definitions of a system in the *Oxford Pocket Dictionary* is 'method, organization, principles of procedure'. In this sense a system can be defined as a method of carrying out a task, an organised way of doing something within a practice. Although each system has its own purpose it can be thought of as a building block which contributes to the total work of the practice. Throughout this book are scattered descriptions of individual systems, such as the repeat prescription card procedure (Chapter 13), finance (Chapters 19 and 20) and feedback (Chapter 15). In this chapter the systems which have crept into general practice piecemeal are brought together. Features which are essential for the successful running of all systems are suggested.

Types of System

For convenience general practice systems can be divided into three types, depending on whether they are concerned primarily with practice routines, with clinical care, or with feedback and monitoring practice activity.

1. Practice Routines

In this category can be placed all those procedures and routines which are necessary because the business of a practice is to provide general medical and other services to its registered patients while at the same time being responsible for its own organisation and finance.

Practice routines include procedures for:

1. Registration and deregistration of patients.
2. Receiving and recording messages.
3. Making appointments.
4. Compiling medical/social records about individual patients.
5. Repeat prescribing.
6. Routine financial transactions.
7. Filing systems.

2. Clinical Care Systems

These systems are those which cater for particular aspects of patient care. They may include systems for:

1. Provision of contraceptive care.
2. Provision of antenatal and postnatal care.
3. Paediatric surveillance.
4. Hypertension screening.
5. Geriatric screening.
6. Surveillance and monitoring of groups of patients who have disorders in common (e.g. diabetes, thyroid problems, hypertension).

3. Feedback: Information Systems

Under this heading fall those systems whose purpose is to provide information about the practice population and practice activities. They include:

1. Characteristics of the practice population: age/sex register.
2. Analysis of morbidity within the practice population: disease register.
3. Analysis of practice workload.
4. Financial analysis.

Examples of Systems

In order to consider factors common to all successful systems, one example of each of these types will be discussed in greater detail.

1. Appointment Systems

The aim of an appointment system is to provide appropriate units of time whereby patients can consult doctors. Patients should have a reasonable choice of time without undue delay and doctors should see a manageable number of patients appropriate to each practitioner and the practice as a whole.

Mr Macawber's remark that with an income of £1, expenditure of £1.0s.6d leads to misery whereas expenditure of 19/6d results in happiness may be applied to appointment systems. A small excess of demand over supply builds up to misery, a small regular surplus of appointments results in happiness all round.

In one author's practice it was decided that the first step in reorganising the appointment system was to find out exactly how many patients were seen over a full year, month by month (to include seasonal variations). With a mid-year list size of 2,013 the figures were:

1983		1984	
July	389	January	494
August	395	February	444
September	471	March	551
October	427	April	411
November	464	May	436
December	436	June	453

Total: 5,371
Average per month: 444

The range was from a low of 389 to a high of 551. However, apart from the highest and lowest months, the other ten fit within 50 plus or minus of the average figure. It was planned, therefore, that each month the average number of appointments (444) plus 10 per cent, i.e. 488 appointments, would be made available. Although these calculations were only concerned with one of the factors involved in running a successful appointment system, the receptionists have subsequently reported that the system has worked much more smoothly since this change was made.

2. Monitoring Patients with Hypertension

In another author's practice, with a large number of middle-aged and elderly patients, it became plain that a considerable amount of consultation time was being taken up by routine blood pressure testing of patients on hypotensive drugs. An extended examination to include weight, urine testing, eye testing and retinal examination was also carried out annually on each hypertensive patient. It was agreed by the partners to introduce a system whereby the practice nurses would take part in the monitoring of this group of patients. The partners met the two nurses concerned in a session over lunch and explained the problem. The nurses were enthusiastic to co-operate and within an hour the procedure and safeguards had been worked out. Agreement was reached, for example, on a standard method of taking and recording the pressure, on the setting of limits of permissible variation in individual patients before referral

back to the doctor, on the setting of intervals between examinations. The agreed procedure was written down and subsequently circulated. At a review three months later the arrangements appeared to be working satisfactorily.

3. Characteristics of the Practice Population: an Age/sex Register

At its simplest the age/sex register is a loose-leaf folder or card index system in which all the patients are grouped according to sex and date of birth. The objective is to enable the practice to know at any one time how many people of a particular age group and sex are registered and who they are. This information has relevance for planning. For example the time and effort spent in screening all patients aged over 70 will be so much greater in a practice with 16 per cent of its population in this category than in one with 6 per cent that the exercise, although worthy, may be impracticable. On the other hand, a predominantly younger practice will have to make different arrangements for giving all its registered pre-school children their boosters when compared with one in a retirement area.

Knowledge of the names and addresses of people in each age group is also the essential prerequisite of all preventive medicine within the practice. Although many practices use the call system which is available for immunisations from health authority computers, many prefer to use their own system, one reason being that when dealing with mobile populations a practice system can be faster and more complete than a centralised one. For other preventive procedures the age/sex register is the only source of organised information.

Keeping the age/sex register accurate and up to date can be a major difficulty. If staff do not see it being used they quickly lose interest — and this can lead to omissions and errors. Certainly comparison between the medical records held, the FPC list, and the age/sex cards in practices which have computerised their practice registers, have shown up major discrepancies.

Essential Features of Practice Systems

Consideration of the three examples described above suggests that systems are much more likely to run smoothly and successfully if certain conditions are met. For example, if the staff cannot see the point of doing something, or there is no agreed procedure, then the system is less likely to work satisfactorily than if the staff are enthusiastic and know what to do.

There are, in fact, a number of principles relating to the organisation of practice activities which are applicable to all businesses, including general practice:

1. Each system should have an objective, be designed for a specific task

One has only to listen to a senior member of staff trying to explain the purpose of an age/sex register to a new member to realise how often doctors ask their staff to do something without explaining the reason for undertaking the task in the first place.

2. Each objective should state the performance to be achieved

For an appointment system the performance might be that all urgent requests are seen the same day and that non-urgent requests should be seen within 48 hours. For hypertensive surveillance it could be that all patients with a history of hypertension should be seen annually for an examination by a doctor and at least once a year by the practice nurse. For an age/sex register the performance could be that the register should be an accurate and up-to-date record of all patients registered with the practice. Without an agreed standard to aim at there is no way of judging whether the system is succeeding or failing.

3. The people who work the system should agree that the task is worthwhile

If the task is thought to be a waste of time, even though the objective is understood, motivation quickly disappears. Such a situation can happen if for example an age/sex register is laboriously maintained but never used.

4. The people who are responsible for running the system should take part in its planning. For established systems they should be encouraged to suggest and make modifications in procedure

It is rare that new systems function perfectly. While partners may be aware that something is not right, it is the people working the system who can best put a finger on what is wrong and who are likely to produce practical suggestions for improvement. The fact that their suggestions are listened to and acted upon increases motivation and a sense of responsibility. 'We do it like this' and 'they told us to do it this way' describe two different worlds in terms of attitudes and management.

5. The procedure used in the system should be written down

This may seem unnecessary in practices where a system is working well and 'everyone knows how to do it'. But people fall ill or retire. Moreover, procedures can be modified by small changes so that over time the system can almost imperceptibly become radically different. A third reason for having a written record of the procedure is that it can be referred to in case of disagreement. Finally, if there is a written record the partners can know what is going on in their practice. It is our experience that in very few practices can the partners describe what their staff actually do.

6. A method of measuring performance should be built into each system

For many practitioners this is the most difficult of the principles to put into practice. Once something is ticking over we tend to assume that everything is going well until confronted with total breakdown. Even then the temptation is to mutter, soldier on, and hope things will improve. The two main reasons for building regular monitoring into a system are that it will pick up inefficiencies early, before crisis point is reached, and that feedback about the system and the fact that it is working well increases the morale and motivation of the people responsible for running it.

For each new system introduced into the practice, decisions have to be made during the planning stage as to what measures shall be taken, whether they should be recorded continuously or whether there should be spot checks, whose responsibility is it to correlate the measures, and to whom the results should be reported.

Conclusion

If the three examples of systems described earlier are examined to discover how well they conform to the 'essential features of practice systems' listed above, both credits and deficiencies will be recognised. It is our belief, based on experience, that one of the most rewarding management activities a practice can undertake is methodically to review the systems in use. The discussion should involve all partners and staff responsible for running each system and should agree how the essential features may be incorporated. This is a lengthy task, not to be rushed. But the benefits in terms of efficiency, morale and motivation can be considerable.

23 THE TRAINING PRACTICE

Over the past decade the number of practices involved in training has increased dramatically. The number of practices recognised for vocational training has doubled in the past five years, and with the advent of mandatory vocational training is unlikely to diminish. A period in general practice is now considered an essential part of the curriculum in most medical schools. Increasingly the training of community nurses, health visitors and social workers involves periods in the community attached to selected practices.

These developments have inevitably affected training practices in various ways. This chapter discusses the benefits and ill-effects which may ensue, and offers guidance on the special points of organisation which are needed within a training practice.

In an established practice, with settled staff and partners, methods and patterns of work have built up over a period of time. The people involved have got to know each other and, it is hoped, have developed a common purpose and identity. They are used to each other. Into this comfortable atmosphere the introduction of a stranger can be a disturbing event. There is potential disruption of routine, of working methods and of relationships. There may on the other hand be positive benefits to the practice with the introduction of new ideas or with a critical eye being turned on what has become too cosy, slack or rigid.

The extent of these effects will depend on the type of visitor, the personality of the individual, the length of time the visitor stays and the extent to which his activities penetrate the organisation. A social work student for a day, a medical student for a week, a health visitor trainee attached for three months, or a medical trainee for a year, will have different effects and repercussions.

Short-term Attachments

These attachments which last from a short visit of a few hours to one of several weeks are of two main types. In the first type the visitor wishes to explore a particular feature of the practice (record systems, computers, premises). Such visits usually involve one member of staff and are made for a specific purpose. It is essential that the purpose of the visit should be clearly defined and that one particular member of staff should be made responsible for looking after the visitor. If such visits become regular or repeated they can become a burden, interfering with practice routine and disrupting the work of the staff members involved. It is necessary to recognise the resentment this may cause and to come to an agreed practice policy involving both partners and staff.

The second type of short-term visitor is usually someone who has little experience or different experience and wishes to increase his/her knowledge of British general practice. A medical student for a fortnight, an American or French doctor for a week, a social work student for one day or week or for a month or two. With this type of visitor, who is likely to be an 'observer' rather than a 'participator', it is also necessary to define the purpose of the visit — both for the practice and the visitor. A timetable, preferably written if more than one person is involved, can be made out so that everyone can know where the visitor is and what they are supposed to be doing. The programme will depend on the visitor and the purpose of the visit. Questions to be answered will be:

(1) Who has overall responsibility for the visitor?
(2) What experience should the programme include?

Responsibility: for day-to-day activities responsibility for the visitor will usually be taken by the practice member of a similar profession, e.g. health visitor for health visitor, practice nurse for practice nurse, doctor for medical student, with the doctors having overall responsibility for what goes on within their practice.

Experience: this will include decisions as to whom the visitor should observe and why. Should they observe office routine, should they be present on home visits or in consultations, should they look at the books, attend staff or partnership meetings? In making these decisions there are some guiding rules which if followed minimise upset to staff and patients.

(1) That persons being observed by the visitor must have agreed to be observed.

(2) That the privacy of patients in the consultation should not be breached unless there are clear reasons for doing so. The visitor

should be introduced and the reasons for the visit explained (albeit briefly) to the patients.

(3) That decisions concerning participation of the visitor in partnership business should be explicitly agreed by all the partners.

(4) That the time and effort taken in entertaining the visitor should be understood by colleagues. Adjustments of practice workload should be made if this is appropriate.

Long-term Attachments

A long-term visitor, although an observer at the beginning of the attachment, is likely to become a participator — the longer the attachment, the greater the participation. Greater participation involves greater penetration of the group activities. It involves relationships with staff and partners which are not just temporary and superficial. It involves relationships with patients. If the visitor is a doctor in training, it involves acceptance by the partnership as a colleague, part of whose training may include knowledge of intimate partnership matters. It is as important that the questions which pertain to a short-term attachment concerning responsibility for the visitor, the purpose of the attachment, and the experience needed should be answered. It is also as important that the 'teachers', whether they be staff or partners, should be willing to teach, should be given time within their workload to teach and that the patients' need for privacy is respected. But the dimension added by time and participation raises further questions, namely:

(1) the effect of trainees on patients;
(2) the effect of trainees on staff;
(3) the effect of trainees on the partners;
(4) the effect of trainees on the practice.

On Patients

(1) The use of the consultation as an opportunity for teaching is one way in which the presence of a trainee directly affects patients. All methods of teaching disturb the normal one-to-one aspect of the consultation. Whether the trainee is an observer, or the trainee conducts the consultation and the trainer is an observer, to the patient this is an abnormal situation, usually unwelcome. The degree of patient displeasure will depend on the

relationship between doctor and patient, the personality and problem of the patient and whether he or she has grown used to the situation in a teaching practice. The use of tape-recorders and video-cameras as a teaching aid is also an intrusion into the patients' privacy — but one which experience shows is rarely resented by patients if they understand the reasons it is being done.

(2) The presence of a trainee affects the continuity of care patients receive. In practices where patients normally see whichever doctor is available, the presence of a trainee adds another possibility of diminishing continuity. Instead of one to two, patients may see any one of three doctors in a two-man partnership. In practices where patients normally see their 'own' doctors, the probability of seing their own doctor, and thus of continuity, is lessened.

(3) The presence of a trainee affects the personal nature of the care patients receive. This is another aspect of loss of continuity. When a practitioner who regularly sees his own patients, and whose patients expect to see him, becomes a trainer the introduction of a trainee may result in the trainer's personal commitment being diminished in the eyes of the patients. They may feel rejected.

On Staff

(1) For staff, particularly staff who have been with the practice a long time, the introduction of a trainee may also be a disturbing event. They may feel that the trainee has no real commitment to 'their practice', that he is a bird of passage. With attachments for a few months, particularly in schemes where trainees are attached to several practices in succession in order to broaden their experience, the staff may scarcely have adjusted to the habits and personality of one trainee, when they are asked to accommodate another.

(2) With a trainee in the practice the workload of staff may increase considerably. In day-to-day practice there is little time for the trainer to explain all the minutiae of practice organisation to each trainee. The majority of questions as they arise will inevitably be dealt with by the staff— where are the forms, when does the blood go to the laboratory and how, when do we get X-ray results? These questions expand into practice policies — who tests the urines, when are swabs taken, how do I best arrange a course of desensitising injections, what is the practice policy for pill checks? Again, unless the trainee is to be eternally bombarding his trainer

with such questions, the staff will answer most of them. They may well find themselves being asked to explain practice policies which they themselves do not understand.

(3) The task of arranging the appointment list for consultations with a trainee largely falls on receptionists. They are responsible for explaining to patients that they will be seeing the trainee rather than their own doctor and will at times have to use diplomacy when exposed to the patients' reactions after seeing 'the new doctor'.

On the Partners

(1) Although the initial impact of a trainee on the way the partners practise will be felt by his trainer, as he sees patients from the other partners their habits also will come under scrutiny. The teacher is aware from the beginning that inevitably his consultations, his methods, diagnostic ability and records will all be under scrutiny. It may only slowly dawn on the other partners that the trainee is forming an opinion of their abilities also. Such realisation can give rise to anxiety and possibly unhappiness between colleagues. The stranger may be looked on as a spy.

(2) This uncertainty may give rise to difficulties within the partnership as to how much the stranger should be allowed to see. There may be disagreements over the trainee's presence at partnership meetings where sensitive matters are discussed. There may be reluctance to open the books.

On the Practice

(1) The overall effect of a long attachment on a practice will inevitably largely depend on the personality and ability of the trainee, and whether this meshes satisfactorily or unsatisfactorily with the practice identity and ability. In addition there are two main considerations. On the one hand, the anxieties and extra work involved for staff and partners will tend to exaggerate and show up any tensions which exist, between partners, between staff, between partners and staff, between patients and practice. On the other hand, the presence of an enquiring stranger within the practice is a potent factor for inducing change. If records are poor, if practice management is faulty, if questions cannot be answered, if gaps are exposed, the stimulus to make changes increases.

(2) Organisation within the practice itself must include accommodation of the stranger. For trainees this increasingly

means a separate consulting room for their use. It means provision of an emergency case, equipment, books. It may also mean advice and help with living accommodation. It means space to park their car.

In summary, the presence of a stranger in the camp will inevitably have effects on a practice and on all those involved. The good effects can be enhanced and the disturbing effects minimised if both staff and partners are aware in advance of the considerations involved. It is equally important that the visitor is aware of the effects his/her presence will have.

PART SEVEN:

THE WIDER WORLD

24 INTERESTS OUTSIDE THE PRACTICE

The family doctor, like other professional people, will almost certainly become involved with interests outside his practice. Some of these will be an inevitable consequence of his being a general practitioner, such as being eligible to vote for his representative on the Local Medical Committee (LMC), whilst others may be an expected duty of the 'village doctor', such as presidency of the village Cricket Club.

In this chapter we shall look at outside interests which are directly related to being a medical practitioner. These have been divided into those which are likely to be done for love and those which are carried out for money.

For Love

The British Medical Association, the Royal College of General Practitioners and the Local Medical Committee are the three medical organisations with which general practitioners are most likely to be involved. They represent the general practitioners' interests in the field of medical politics, training, continuing education and research. All three have a local structure, which means that the general practitioner can seek advice or participate in the organisation at a local level. In the case of the British Medical Association, the local structure depends upon the local division. The Royal College of General Practitioners has faculties at a regional level adminstered by a Faculty Board. The Local Medical Committee operates over an area similar to that administered by the Family Practitioner Committee and, in some cases, even has district subdivisions so that individual general practitioners may refer to their local district committee of the LMC. The central body for Local Medical Committees is the General Medical Services Committee.

Although the Royal College of General Practitioners, the British Medical Association and the General Medical Services Committee have interests in common in the field of general practice, their functions are mainly complementary, and their membership is obtained in different ways.

The Local Medical Committee

All general practitioners in contract with a Family Practitioner Committee have a vote in electing their representative to serve on the Local Medical Committee. Thus, the LMC is the only truly representative body of all the general practitioners working in the National Health Service. At the local level, it is the responsibility of the LMC to watch over the interests of its members and to negotiate the settlement of local medical difficulties. It is also responsible for appointing the medical members of the Family Practitioner Committee and its sub-committees. It thus has considerable influence over medical administration in the general practitioner's area. In particular, it appoints members to the local

Table 24.1 Local Medical Committee Agenda

1. Apologies for absence.
2. Minutes of the previous meeting.
3. Matters arising from the minutes.
4. Report on the Annual Conference of Representatives of the LMCs.

5a. Election of member of FPC dispensing sub-committee.

5b. Election of a member on North Wessex Disablement Advisory Committee

5c. Election of a member to the Ophthalmic Service Committee. (Deputies may be appointed for all these representatives.)

6. Appointment of practice nurses (see enclosed memorandum).
7. Storage of drugs in surgeries; to receive a memorandum from the police.
8. To receive reports from representatives of:
   a) The regional medical committee.
   b) The GMS committee.
   c) The Area Health Care Planning Team (mental illness).
9. To receive accounts for the year ended 31 March.
10. District sub-committee reports.
11. Matters arising from circulars received.
    a) GMSC circulars.
       i) Review Body report.
       ii) Cameron Fund Limited.
    b) DHSS circulars.
       i) Senior management education and training.
       ii) Prescription charges (revised forms FP57).
12. Mileage allowances for attendances at courses.
13. New forms FP19 (temporary residence).
14. Payments for loss or damage of oxygen equipment.
15. Trainees, allowances for additional car.
16. Remuneration of general medical practitioners (Review Body increases).
17. Any other business.
18. Date of next meeting.

Signed, Clerk to the Committee.

Medical Practices Committee which itself appoints doctors to single-handed practices, to the Medical Services Committee which is responsible for investigating complaints made against family doctors, and to the Local Obstetric Committee which, amongst other things, is responsible for the appointment of general practitioners to the obstetric list. A typical LMC agenda is illustrated in Table 24.1. Elections to the Local Medical Committee are on a constituency basis. Each general practitioner has his own elected representative member. He is, therefore, able to raise individual problems directly with his own representative.

Each year each local medical committee sends a number of its members to represent it at the annual Conference of Local Medical Committees and each year several medical committees together elect a member to serve on the General Medical Services Committee (GMSC). The GMSC is the executive of the conference of LMCs. It negotiates with the Department of Health and Social Security on the terms and conditions of service for general practitioners working within the National Health Service as the sole representative of all general practitioners. Members of the GMSC are not necessarily members of the BMA.

The LMCs are financed by statutory levy on every general practitioner in their area. In addition, there is a voluntary levy on general practitioners for activities not specified by statute and for the General Medical Services Defence Trust — the general practitioners' fighting fund.

The British Medical Association

The British Medical Association is a voluntary association with members in all branches of the medical profession, both in and out of the National Health Service. Its prime objectives, as stated in the Memorandum of Association, are 'to promote the medical and allied sciences, and to maintain the honour and interests of the medical profession'.

It is both a registered company, limited by guarantee, and an independent trade union listed under the Trade Union and Labour Relations Act 1974. Four of its standing committees representing the Hospital Medical Service, General Practice, Junior Hospital Doctors and Community Medicine are recognised by the Secretary of State for Social Services as sole negotiators with the Department of Health and Social Services on all matters relating to their respective branches of the profession.

In addition to its trade union function, the BMA has a range of committees to deal with specific aspects of medical practice. There is a Private Practice Committee which, among other things, negotiates fees for its members with non-NHS bodies including other government departments. There is an Ethical Committee which considers a very wide range of matters from the use of torture in interrogation, and the confidentiality of medical data, to disputes between individual members of the profession. The Board of Science and Education provides an authoritative professional response to many matters of public interest. On behalf of the Association it brings together the views of all branches of the profession on such matters as the age of consent, seat-belts and abortions. It also advises on the library at BMA House, distributes awards and prizes, and arranges the annual clinical meetings of the association. There are many other committees such as those for the Armed Forces, Occupational Health and Medical Charities. The *British Medical Journal* is highly regarded world-wide and is free to members.

At a local level, the division is a forum for members of all branches of the profession and encourages interchange and understanding between them in both the medical and political fields. The regional secretariat provides a 'trouble-shooting' back-up to the shop-steward activities of the Divisional Honorary Secretary. All divisions elect representatives to the Annual Representative Meeting. In this way they have a voice in the decision-making of the Association, as the Representative Body is the policy-making body of the Association and the Council, its executive, is bound by the decisions of the Representative Body. It therefore behoves every general practitioner to be a member of the Association in order to play his or her full part as a responsible member of the medical profession.

The Royal College of General Practitioners

The Royal College of General Practitioners was founded as the College of General Practitioners in 1952. Its membership has grown to approximately 10,000 and a high proportion of new entrants to general practice sit its membership examination. Whilst the other two organisations concern themselves with representation of doctors' interests in the political field and the provision of supporting services the RCGP is primarily concerned with raising the standard of general practice through education, improvements in practice organisation, and by encouraging research. Many members have played an active part in the larger research projects of the College, one of the best known being the Oral Contraception Study. The RCGP publishes a monthly journal of general practice, the *Journal of the Royal College of General Practitioners*, and a growing list of occasional papers relevant to general practice. Like the BMA subscription the RCGP subscription is a tax-allowable practice expense.

The College is organised in regional faculties, each being administered by a Faculty Board. Members and associates are allotted to the faculty within whose area they reside, although they may elect to change to another faculty if it is more convenient. Most faculties hold regular meetings throughout their areas. Local education and research groups may be formed and most post-graduate centres have a College representative.

Because of its interest in medical education, the College is particularly active in all vocational training schemes. Where these are in operation the College tutor and the course organiser are usually to be found working together. The book *The Future General Practitioner, Learning and Teaching* (1972) was one of the first attempts to analyse and describe the content of general practice. Not surprisingly it is considered essential reading for all those interested in teaching general practice.

Other Organisations

In most areas of the country there are established local medical societies which play an active part in the professional life of the locality. Nowadays many of these hold their meetings in post-graduate medical centres. For a small subscription they usually provide an interesting medical and social programme. A local society often provides a doctor new to the area with a forum where he may meet colleagues in both general practice and hospital practice.

Professional Representative Activities

Most professions have a complicated structure for self-regulation and for representation at various levels. The need for a strong organisation within general practice is necessary not only to negotiate pay and conditions of service but increasingly to represent the viewpoint and interests of general practice at local, regional, national and international level. There are a large number of appointments available (summarised as a list in Section 2 of this chapter). For most of these appointments expenses only are received, so that if a partner becomes involved in committee work it must be with the prior agreement of the remaining partners in order to avoid friction. We have no doubt however that in order to maintain standards within general practice and provide the resources necessary to do so, strong and capable professional representation is essential.

For Money

Medical earnings from all sources inside and outside the practice are usually paid into the common partnership pool. Hence the partners' agreement to the acceptance of outside appointments is essential. A clear agreement as to who gets the money must be made before the appointment is accepted. This should include agreement on superannuation and other benefits.

Clinical Work in Hospitals and Health Authority Clinics

For doctors with special interests and skills the opportunity exists to do sessional work in hospitals and health authority clinics. Most appointments are currently paid at the clinical assistant grade but new appointments should be made at the hospital practitioner grade which properly recognises special skill. Whilst such work inevitably takes the doctor away from his general practice patients, it often benefits his practice in that he is able to maintain a high standard of expertise in his chosen field, and this often benefits both his patients and his partners in the practice.

Care must be taken that pursuing an interest does not cost the partnership money. For example, the doctor may work in an Health Authority family planning clinic on a sessional basis and find that he does all the family planning work for the patients of his practice at a relatively small fee; whereas if he had provided a practice family planning service, the total reimbursement under the FPC contraceptive service would have been much greater. On the other hand, work in child health clinics, whilst often reducing a practice's income from the immunisations, usually will result in a net financial gain to the partnership from the sessional payments.

Work in additional clinical fields provides useful and interesting contacts. It is this aspect rather than money earned which is the main attraction to many general practitioners. The doctor's primary commitment must be to his practice and patients. Such sessional work cannot in our opinion exceed more than five half-days without loss of continuity of patient care.

School Medical Officers

Many practices provide medical services for residential schools within the practice area. It is common for such schools to retain the services of a particular practitioner as the 'school doctor'. In that case, not only will he be responsible for the day-to-day health of the pupils and staff (who are usually registered on his 'medical list') but he will also be called upon to carry out a large number of duties outside the National Health Service. These are mostly in the field of preventive medicine and include the following:

(a) Advising the headmaster or governing body in matters of health.

(b) Liaison with house masters and reporting to them or to the school matron fitness for activities of individual pupils.

(c) Epidemiological control within the school.

(d) Reporting annually on the health of the school and the sanitary condition of the premises. It is usual for the medical officer to be available to inspect drainage, sanitary provision, the dormitories, studies and common-rooms, lighting, cleanliness and heating of classrooms; also water, milk, and food supplies and kitchen hygiene.

(e) The administration of the sanatorium and direction of nursing staff duties.

(f) Admission examinations of pupils, periodic medical examinations and examinations when a pupil leaves the school.

(g) The proper keeping of medical records and regulations.

(h) The control of disinfection and hygienic disposal of refuse.

(i) Reports to parents or guardians.

(j) Medical examinations for the services, universities, employment medical advisory service, sub aqua clubs, etc.

(k) Correspondence with university medical officers.

These duties command a special fee, usually paid termly. Special surgeries are commonly held at the school for the convenience of staff and pupils.

The Medical Officers of Schools Association is an organisation which represents doctors working with schools. It arranges national meetings about topics of interest to school doctors. It also publishes the *Handbook of School Health* (16th Edition, 1984), a very useful guide for school doctors and all others who are concerned in the health and welfare of young people. The Association also publishes regular news letters.

From time to time, the Medical Officers of Schools Association and the BMA publish a recommended scale of fees for school medical officers. It must be emphasised that no fee can be claimed for any duty which is covered by the National Health Service Act 1946, but fees are due for the additional duties outlined above. In 1984 the Medical Officers of Schools Association approved a recommended fee of £12.60 per pupil per year. The recommended BMA rate is higher. It should be noted that the Association of Governing Bodies of Public Schools has advised that 'all schools should from time to time review the fees payable to part-time medical officers to ensure that they are properly remunerated'. Since no two schools are identical, the scale referred to above should be taken as a guide for negotiating the appropriate fee in each individual case.

Other Appointments

In any area, the scope for additional appointments for doctors is considerable. Doctors who work on a part-time basis to service the needs of various government departments are usually termed Treasury Medical Officers. They may advise government departments on the fitness of prospective employees, the prognosis in staff who are sick, and on whether or not staff should be retired prematurely on health grounds. Main regional centres require police surgeons, and factories large and small are required by the Factory Act to have a named medical adviser.

Fees for all such appointments are negotiated and recommended by the Private Practice Committee of the BMA. However, doctors are always advised to negotiate an appropriate fee in the light of the expected work. For example, a small factory producing heavy industrial products may require a good deal more time than a larger light industrial concern.

Writing, Lecturing and Broadcasting

For a few doctors these activities constitute a major source of income. For many more an occasional contribution will earn some pin-money. There are opportunities in national magazines and journals, as a contributor to a book, and particularly at present in local broadcasting.

Teaching

Many doctors enjoy teaching. Opportunities now exist in general practice for taking part in the undergraduate teaching programmes of most medical schools, in training future general practitioners through vocational training schemes, and by acting as a general practitioner trainer. At present (1984) well over 1,000 general practitioners are involved in teaching within their own practices.

In addition a smaller number are employed as course organisers. A course organiser is paid at the same rate as a trainer. As well as being closely involved with a vocational training scheme he (or she) will frequently help in selection of trainers, in running trainers' groups, and be closely connected with the postgraduate tutors at the local postgraduate centre.

Within each region there now exists a Regional General Practice Advisory Service which acts as an academic support system. The Regional Adviser, a general practitioner in active practice, is responsible for organising the service — usually supported by one or two assistant advisers. These appointments are University appointments and attract sessional payments at the top of the clinical consultant scale.

Although those who take part generally do so from sheer enthusiasm, increased income can result from these activities. Medical schools pay an honorarium to the general practitioner supervisors, while general practitioner trainers receive the trainer's grant at the rate of £3,160 a year (1984) for the time a trainee is placed with them. The recommendation of the Joint Committee on Postgraduate Training for General Practice is that trainers should set aside at least two sessions per week for teaching their trainee and in additions should participate regularly in the local trainers' workshop. Course organisers are paid the same sum annually as general practitioner trainers, but do not have a trainee attached to them in their practices. Doctors teaching at vocational training or other postgraduate courses are entitled to a lecture fee for each session given. All this represents a considerable change from the situation which existed only a very few years ago. It reflects the importance now attached to training for general practice.

References and Further Reading

Handbook of School Health. Issued by Medical Officers of Schools Association, 16th Edition (London: MTP 1984).

History of the British Medical Association 1832-1932. Compiled by E.M. Little (London: BMA, 1932).

History of the British Medical Association 1932-1981. Elston Grey-Turner and S.M. Sutherland. (London: B.M.A. 1982).

Journal of the Royal College of General Practitioners, 27 (1977), no. 184. This is the 'Silver Jubilee number' and commemorates the 25th anniversary of the founding of the (then) College of General Practitioners on 19 November 1952.

Vaughan, P. *Doctors' Commons* (London: Heinemann, 1959).

Chapter 24: Section 2

A summary of the positions to which general practitioners may be elected or appointed within the Health Service and to bodies which represent the profession at a national or international level. This is by no means a complete list as a look at the annual GMSC or RCGP Council report will show.

1. *Local and district representation*

on the Local Medical Committee (LMC): elected by colleagues
on the RCGP Faculty Board: elected by members of the faculty
on the District Management Team: elected by the LMC
on the Unit Management Team: elected by the LMC
on the District Health Authority: appointed by the Regional Health Authority after consultation with local medical bodies
on the Family Practitioner Committee: appointed by the Secretary of State after nomination by local medical bodies

2. *Regional representation*

Although membership of the Regional Health Authority is by appointment by the Secretary of State from a list of practitioners nominated by local medical bodies, other regional appointments are normally filled by direct election by the profession itself.

Advising the Regional Health Authority are:
the Regional Medical Advisory Committee
the Regional Manpower Committee
the Regional Postgraduate Education Committee
the Regional Locally Organised Research Committee
the Regional General Practice Specialty Committee
the Regional General Practice Education Committee

3. *National representation*

on the General Medical Service Committee: election is by colleagues on a regional or a national basis
on the Council of the RCGP: election is by college members either nationally or by faculty

on the Council of the British Medical Association: election is by BMA members on a regional and national basis at the annual meeting of the Representative Body
on the General Medical Council: election is by national ballot of the whole profession

4. *International representation*

A few general practitioners may be elected or nominated to serve on international organisations which include:
the European Union of General Practitioners (UEMO)
the Societas Internationalis Medicine Generalis (SIMG)
the World Organisation of National Colleges and Academies (WONCA)

25 THE SETTING: THE PRACTICE WITHIN THE HEALTH SERVICE

Diversity within a small area is a characteristic of Britain. Visitors used to the Rockies, the Plains or the Veldt are surprised how quickly they pass from town to country, to isolated communities, and back again. General practice reflects this diversity. Within fifty miles of any city the whole range of different types of practice can be found: the large group practice, the small practice, the one-man practice; the urban practice where all the patients may live within a half-mile radius, the rural practice where the practice area is commonly one hundred square miles or more; practices in health centres, in adapted or purpose-built premises, branch surgeries in the back room of the village shop. Each type of practice, each location, has its own particular problems and its own compensations.

There is, however, one factor common to all. Each general practitioner who works in the National Health Service in England and Wales has a contract with a Family Practitioner Committee or Committee acting on behalf of the Department of Health and Social Security. In this contract (form FP16) he/she agrees to be bound by 'the terms of service for the time being in that area'. In Scotland and Northern Ireland the position is different. The differences, which mainly involve the organisation of the NHS in these parts, are outlined in later sections of this chapter.

Terms of Service

The terms of service 'for the time being' are based on paragraph 13 of the first schedule of the NHS Regulations 1974 which states that

> a doctor shall render to his patients all necessary and appropriate personal medical services of the type usually provided by general medical practitioners. He shall do so at his practice premises or, if the condition of his patient so requires, elsewhere in his practice area. Such services include arrangements for referring patients as necessary to the hospital and specialist

services, the general ophthalmic services, and advice to take advantage of the local authority services. Except in an emergency this paragraph shall not impose an obligation on the doctor to provide maternity medical service unless he has undertaken to do so.

This wording, by virtue of its flexibility, has survived inquiries, a Royal Commission and several National Service Acts.

Organisation of the National Health Service

The way in which the National Health Service was run in England and Wales between April 1974 and April 1982 was laid down in 1972 in a publication from the DHSS called *Management Arrangements for the Reorganised National Health Service.* The framework of the organisation, as quoted from this publication, was planned as follows:

(a) There are to be *Area* Health Authorities (AHA) — including some Area Health Authorities (Teaching) (AHA(T)) with particular medical and dental teaching responsibilities, accountable to *Regional* Health Authorities (RHA), who are in turn accountable to the *Secretary of State* for the effectiveness and efficiency of the services provided.

(b) These AHAs are to be coterminous geographically with the new local authorities (counties and metropolitan districts) which are to be set up outside London, and with the present London Boroughs or combinations of London Boroughs.

(c) Each AHA is to be required by statute to set up a *Family Practitioner Committee* (FPC) to administer the contracts of practitioners.

(d) There is to be statutory provision for the recognition of *professional advisory machinery,* from which RHAs, AHAs and FPCs will draw advice.

(e) *Community Health Councils* (CHC) are to be established to represent the views of the public to the AHAs.

The paper went on to lay down the administrative structure at each level and the roles and responsibilities of all the different people involved (e.g. Regional Treasurer, Area Administrator, District Pharmaceutical Officer, Area Chief Ambulance Officer).

Figure 25.1: Organisation of the National Health Service 1 April 1974 to 1 April 1982 in England and Wales

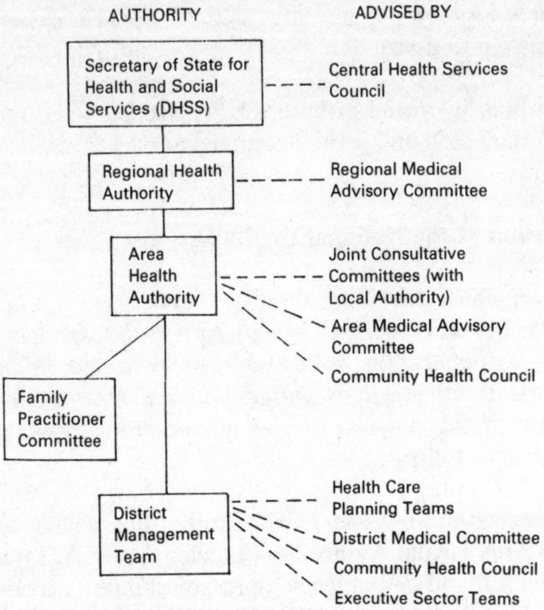

Both the structure itself and the language in which it is described are complicated. The organisation described above became operational on 1 April 1974. The main features of the organisation are shown in Figure 25.1.

This structure was instituted in April 1974, but shortly after its introduction opinions were expressed that there were too many layers of management. In view of this and other areas of controversy the Government set up a Royal Commission in 1975 with the following terms of reference:

> to consider in the interests of both the patients and of those who work in the National Health Service the best use and management of the financial and manpower resources of the National Health Service.

The Commission reported on 18 July 1979. It put forward a number of proposals including the possibility of abolishing the Area level of management and setting up new District Health

Authorities. The Government published its initial reactions as a consultative paper called *Patients First* in December 1979. With some amendments the suggested new structure was agreed between the profession and the Government and published as a Health Circular in July 1980 (HC(80)8). It came into operation on 1 April 1982. Further legislation in 1984 established Family Practitioner Committees as free-standing bodies responsible to government, with chairmen appointed by government. This change is due to be implemented on 1 April 1985. The present structure is as shown in Figure 25.2, but in the current political climate it is doubtful how long it will be given to settle down before further changes are introduced. At the time of writing the Government is due to announce its decision whether or not to introduce the appointment of 'managers' into the NHS (as proposed in the Griffiths report). Griffiths suggested that a general manager should be appointed for each level in each unit, district and region throughout England and Wales, topped off by a Health Services Supervisory Board to advise the Secretary of State for Social Services on the 'strategic direction of the Health Services'. Time will tell whether this would actually benefit the delivery of care to patients or whether it is another expensive and disruptive waste of time.

When he first enters practice, the relationship between Health Care Planning Teams, District Managment Teams (DMT) and Unit Management Teams (UMT) are unlikely to worry the young general practitioner with his mortgage, his new practice and young family, but the work of these committees directly affects all general practitioners. They do this by making policy decisions which determine the local allocation of available resources. These decisions directly influence the working conditions of all general practitioners in the district.

Regional Health Authority

In England there are 14 Regional Health Authorities. They are accountable to the Secretary of State for the effectiveness and efficiency of the health services provided in their regions. They are responsible for co-ordinating strategic plans and for resource allocations to districts. Each Regional Health Authority consists of a chairman (appointed by the Secretary of State) and a number of

Figure 25.2: Organisation of the National Health Service in England and Wales from 1 April 1985

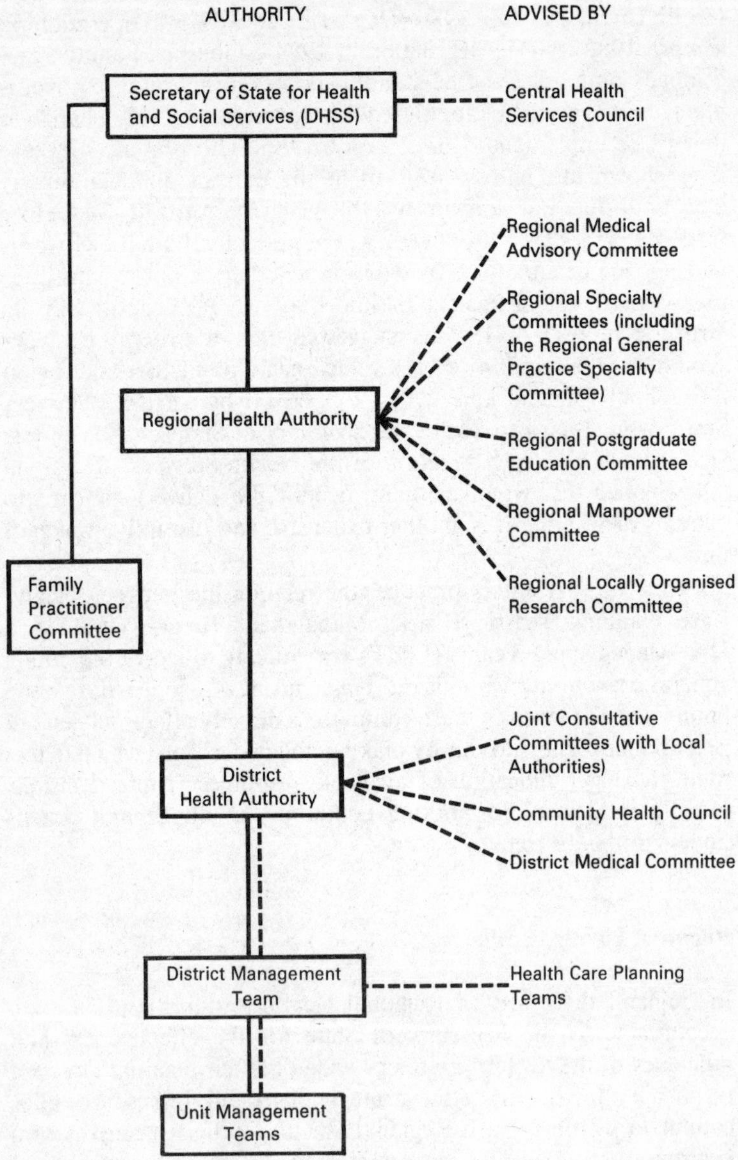

officers (e.g. Regional Administrator, Regional Treasurer, Regional Medical Officer). It is advised by a number of professional committees.

District Health Authority

Each DHA is responsible for the planning, development and management of health services in its district within national and regional guidelines. Most districts contain between 200,000 and 500,000 people. The appointment of members of the DHA is as follows:

Chairman, appointed by the Secretary of State
12 members appointed by the RHA
- one hospital consultant
- one general practitioner
- one nurse, midwife or health visitor
- one university nominee
- one member nominated by the trade unions
- up to seven 'generalist members'

4 members appointed by local authorities

It will be appreciated that in such a body which determines which local services shall be developed and which cut, and decides how many hundreds of thousands of pounds shall or shall not be spent on equipment and staff, in hospitals or in the community, the single general practitioner member has a considerable responsibility.

District Management Team

The District Management Team is responsible for the day-to-day running, of all the NHS services in its district, and for advising the DHA on future planning. This includes capital projects in hospitals and in the community. It includes agreeing a list of priorities for changing the service offered, such as running one service down or extending another. It includes decisions on a range of subjects from the reimbursement of a psychiatric nurse whose coat has been damaged to whether a new hospital should be built.
The members of the District Management Team are as follows:

(1) One hospital specialist.
(2) One general practitioner.
(3) The District Community Physician.
(4) The District Nursing Officer.
(5) The District Administrator.
(6) The District Finance Officer.

Of the six members there are four 'permanent' appointments (finance officer, administrator, nursing officer and community physician); of the three doctors on the District Management Team two are clinicians.

The general practitioner and the hospital specialist on the District Management Team are usually elected by the District Medical Committee from among their own members. This committee, the District Medical Committee, usually has between 12 and 16 members. It is composed of hospital specialists and general practitioners in equal numbers. In some districts, there is a representative of the dentists and other professional workers within the Health Service on this committee, as well as doctors representing a special interest or group. The general practitioner members of the District Medical Committee are themselves elected by their Local Medical Committee. In some districts the profession has decided to disband the District Medical Committee. When this has happened clinical members are usually appointed directly by the Medical Executive and the Local Medical Committee. As will be seen in the section on 'negotiations'. Local Medical Committees have a medico-political function but it is also their responsibility to appoint representatives to the many committees involved in running the Health Service at AHA and district level.

The District Management Team is itself served by Unit Management Teams representing major interests such as the District Hospital, the Community, or Mental Illness. In addition it takes advice from *Health Care Planning Teams.* These are set up by the DHA or DMT to look into the requirements of special groups. There may be a team for child care, another for services to the elderly. There may be a third to look into the running of the hospital transport system.

The Family Practitioner Committee

Although the previous section may seem to many to be of only theoretical interest, the one part of the Health Service organisation with which all general practitioners come in close contact throughout their professional careers is the Family Practitioner Commitee. It is to this Committee that the general practitioner applies to be appointed as a principal in general practice. It is with this Committee that he signs his contract.

The Family Practitioner Committee is currently (1984) an agent of the DHA. Its powers are delegated to it by statute. It administers the Health Service arrangements, not only of general practitioners but also of the opticians, pharmacists and dentists who work within the Health Service in the community as independent contractors. From 1 April 1985 each FPC will become a free-standing authority in its own right, responsible directly to the DHSS.

For the general practitioner the FPC is the direct point of contact with the administration of the Health Service. For many general practitioners who are not involved in committee work it may be their only point of contact. It is the FPC which appoints him as a principal. It is the FPC which pays him. It is through the FPC that a general practitioner receives the medical records of patients when they sign on with him; it is to the FPC that he returns these records when patients leave or die.

The Family Practitioner Committee is the direct successor to the body known before the 1974 reorganisation as the Executive Council. (This explains why the numbers of many forms in use in practice are prefixed by EC. More recent ones are prefixed by FP.) The appointment of the members of the FPC are currently made (1984) as follows:

By the	— District Health Authority	11 members
	— Local Authority	4 members
	— Local Medical Committee	8 members (7 general medical practitioners, 1 ophthalmic medical practitioner)
	— Local Dental Committee	3 members
	— Local Pharmaceutical Committee	2 members
	— Local Optical Committee	2 members

So that, of the 30 members, 15 are appointed by the professions and 15 are laymen. The chairman is at present (1984) elected by the FPC from among its own members.

The areas and population served by different Family Practitioner Committees vary enormously, the smallest being Powys with a population of 100,000 – the largest being Kent with a population of 1,490,000.

Medical Practices Committee

The size of population and the number of practitioners in any one area are governed by many factors. In terms of cost of living, quality of life, the availabilty of good concerts, theatres and schools, each general practitioner will have his own priorities. But some parts of the country are more attractive to a larger number of general practitioners than other parts. In one area there may be an average of 1,600 patients to each general practitioner, in another there may be 3,000. In deciding to appoint a doctor to a practice the FPC is governed by the recommendations of the Medical Practices Committee. This is a national committee which, among its other functions, classifies each locality into one of four different categories:

(1) *Designated areas*: which are under-doctored and to which doctors are encouraged to go by various grants and payments (see Chapter 8). Average list size in a designated area is over 2,500 patients per doctor.

(2) *Open areas*: in which the number of doctors is below the recommended number. In these areas a general practitioner can usually 'put up his plate', but he attracts no special allowances. Average list size in an open area is 2,100-2,500 patients per doctor.

(3) *Intermediate areas*: in which the total number of general practitioners is considered adequate. Usually a general practitioner can only enter practice in an intermediate area if another general practitioner retires. Average list size in an intermediate area is 1,700-2,200 patients per doctor.

(4) *Closed (restricted) areas*: in which the number of patients per doctor is well below the national average. Close scrutiny is given to the necessity of appointing a further general practitioner if one retires. Average list size in a closed area is less than 1,700 patients per doctor.

The Medical Practices Committee meets in London on two days each week. There are nine members appointed by the Secretary of State of whom one is a lay member, one is a barrister, and seven are general practitioners. In deciding whether an additional doctor may be appointed or not in a particular district, the Medical Practices Committee does not rely on rigid criteria of average list size alone. They may exercise their discretion to take account of other factors such as the age of the doctors in the district and in the practice, the number of temporary residents seen or the number of outside appointments held. Many other considerations besides type of area and size of population influence their decision.

Negotiations Between the Profession and the Government

Alteration of the Schedules of the NHS Regulations is by Act of Parliament. Alterations in the Red Book are made by negotiation between representatives of the profession and the DHSS. Amendments to the Red Book, which is discussed in greater detail in Chapter 16, are also made following recommendations of the Review Body — if these are agreed by both Government and the profession.

The Review Body itself was set up following the recommendations of the Royal Commission on Doctors' and Dentists' Remuneration in 1960. The main aim was to avoid recurrent disputes about remuneration by establishing an impartial body which would recommend just levels of payment after hearing evidence from both Government and the profession. The Review Body is free to obtain additional information from whatever source it wishes. It is free to decide its own methods of work, the periods that its recommendations should cover, and how often to undertake reviews. There are seven members and a chairman. In practice in each of the past six years there has been one main review (published in the Spring) supplemented by interim reviews when the need arose.

In addition to this formal review machinery, direct negotiations between the profession and the Department of Health and Social Security occur at regular monthly meetings. The general practitioners who negotiate on behalf of the profession are appointed annually by the *General Medical Services Committee* from among its members. The GMSC currently (1984) has *80* members composed of elected and appointed representatives. The majority of members (42) are general practitioners who are elected by Local Medical Committees throughout the country. A further six are elected annually by the conference of Representatives of Local Medical Committees.

Local Medical Committees in turn are composed of general practitioners, each of whom has been elected by fellow practitioners in his practice district. So when it negotiates with the Government on terms and conditions of service the General Medical Services Committee represents the interests of every general practitioner in the country, whether or not he be a member of the BMA, RCGP, MPU or any other organisation. Because the BMA is the only negotiating body for general practitioners recognised by the Government, however, a typical British compromise has resulted in the GMSC being recognised as a 'craft' committee within the BMA although some of its members may not be members of the Association.

The NHS in Scotland

Although in the main the fees, allowances, terms and conditions of service are the same for general practitioners throughout Great Britain, the health services in Scotland have always operated under separate NHS Acts. In 1978 the various NHS Acts since 1947, including the NHS (Scotland) Act 1972 which corresponds to the Act which reorganised the NHS in England and Wales in 1974, were consolidated under the National Health Service (Scotland) Act 1978.

Patients first, the consultative paper on the structure and management of the NHS issued by the Government in 1979, applied only to England and Wales — but a similar paper was later issued by the Scottish Home and Health Department. Reorganisation was supposed to come into effect on 1 April 1982 (as in England and Wales). In the event, partly because of differences between the structure of the Health Service in Scotland and England since 1974, discussions were prolonged. Suddenly in November 1983 the SHHD announced that rather than setting up authorities at District level all Districts which already existed in Scotland would be scrapped. To date (1984), therefore, the structure remains largely as it was established ten years ago.

In the 1974 reorganisation 15 Health Boards were established in Scotland. These Boards are directly responsible to the Scottish Home and Health Department. Their responsibilities are broadly those which are carried out by Regional and District Health Authorities in England and Wales. The Common Services Agency, which directly administers the Blood Transfusion Service and the Ambulance Service, provides services under the Scottish Home and Health Department for all Health Boards.

Each Health Board delegates administration concerning primary care to a General Medical Practitioner Committee which is composed of equal numbers of lay and medical members together with a lay chairman.

In contrast to the position in England and Wales where general practitioners have contracts with Family Practitioner Committees, each general practitioner in Scotland contracts his or her services to one or more Health Boards.

The medical advisory structure in Scotland is complex. The relationship between the main administrative levels and their advisory committees is shown in Figure 25.3. It will be noted that each Health Board is advised by its Area Medical Committee, a University Liaison Committee and by Local Health Councils. The Area Medical Committee consists of representatives of all Divisions within the Area. Each Area Medical Committee has a subcommittee for general practitioners (which usually has the same membership as the LMC) and most have subcommittees for other specialties.

In addition to advising its Health Board each Area Medical Committee is represented on the National Medical Consultative Committee. This Committee, which includes members from Royal Colleges and Universities, has eleven specialty subcommittees. It is the function of the National Medical Consultative Committee (together with the National Consultative Committees of other professions working in the Health Service) to advise the Scottish Health Services Planning Council on matters of policy in relation to clinical provision. The Planning Council in turn advises the Scottish Home and Health Department.

One major difference between the organisation of the service in England and Wales is that in Scotland no clinician takes a direct part in local management decisions unless he is appointed to a Health Board by the Secretary of State. In England and Wales a general practitioner and hospital specialist are elected by their colleagues to be members of the District Management Team. In this way, clinicians in England and Wales are directly involved in planning and management decisions.

Figure 25.3

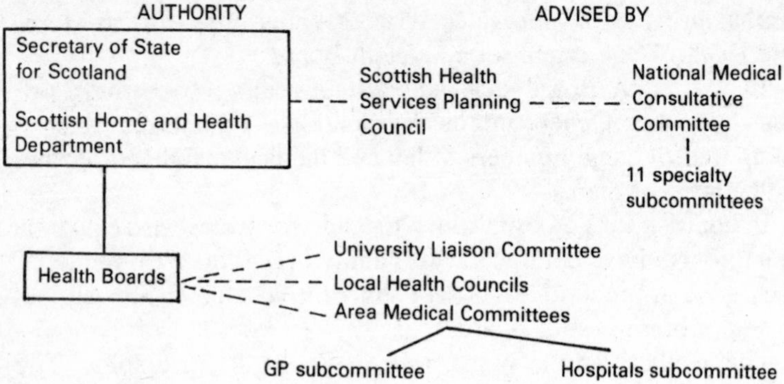

The NHS in Northern Ireland

In Northern Ireland the administration of the Health Service differs from that found in both Scotland and in England and Wales. The main difference is that in Northern Ireland the Health Service and Social Services Departments are integrated at all levels.

In common with the other parts of the United Kingdom, Northern Ireland has recently been convulsed by reorganisation. Prior to 1983 it was administered under a separate Act — the Health and Social Services (Northern Ireland) Order 1972. Following consultations through 1979 and 1980 the Secretary of State issued a statement of the changes to be made (Circular HSS(P)1/81 The Structure and Management of Health and Personal Social Services in Northern Ireland).

Although these changes were meant to be implemented on 1 April 1982 it was not until 1 April 1983 that three of the Health Boards put them into effect and at the time of writing the fourth (Eastern) is still embroiled in discussions.

Organisation not in dispute is as follows: there are four boards called Health and Social Services Boards responsible for administering, planning, monitoring and co-ordinating health and social services within their areas. They are formed on a geographical basis (Western, Southern, Northern and Eastern). They are responsible directly to the Secretary of State for Northern Ireland, and their chairmen and vice-chairmen are appointed directly by him. As in Scotland there are no Family Practitioner Committees. Each general practitioner is in contract with a Board. Responsibility for the day-to-day running of family practitioner services is in the hands of a Central Services Agency acting on behalf of all four Health and Social Services Boards.

Until the 1983/4 reorganisation there were seventeen Districts (each responsible to a Board); each District possessed a planning committee (the District Executive Committee) which had statutory recognition. The composition of the District Executive Committee was as follows:

1. one administrator (District Administrator)
2. one nurse (District Nursing Officer)
3. one clinician (consultant or general practitioner)
4. one social services officer (District Social Services Officer)
5. one community physician (District Community Physician)

Reorganisation resulted in the abolition of Districts and their replacement by a number of Units each supported by a Unit Management Group. It was also suggested that each advisory team should contain a general practitioner and a finance officer. The position is still fluid.

Summing Up

This chapter opened by pointing out the differences between practices, between practices in the same town, between practices in different locations. The rest of the chapter has shown that notwithstanding this diversity and regional variations each practitioner in the Health Service works within the same broad framework.

Further Reading

Management Arrangements for the Reorganised Health Service (London: HMSO, 1972).

Marks, J. *The Conference of Local Medical Committees and its Executive: An Historical Review* (London: General Medical Services Defence Trust, 1979).

Stevens, R. *Medical Practice in Modern England* (New Haven, Conn.: Yale University Press, 1966).

Royal Commission on the National Health Service HMSO London 1979 (Cmnd. 7615).

Levitt, R. and Wall, A. *The Reorganized National Health Service,* 3rd edition (London: Croom Helm, 1984)

DHSS. *Patients First,* (London: HMSO, 1979).

NHS Management Inquiry Report (Griffiths Report) (London: DHSS, 1983).

26 CONCLUSION: LOOKING AT A PRACTICE

There are many different ways of looking at a practice. In the first chapter we described the variety among practices in terms of people, places, provision of services, premises, partners, and the doctors' personality.

From the viewpoint of a young doctor looking for a practice he or she will be more interested in seeing how well the practice matches his or her own preferences. Further discussion on this subject, together with a check list can be found in Appendix I.

When an established practitioner looks at his own practice, however, he will do so from a different angle. Usually he will be trying to judge how well it is performing and how it may be improved. In this chapter we present some of the principles underlying practice management and suggest ways in which signs and symptoms of good and poor management may be recognised.

The Aims of Management

The overall aim of management is to run an efficient business. The problem of defining management thus is that many practitioners relate efficiency to inhumanity. They see an unhealthy regard for money competing with their caring role. In answer we would point out that in common usage the word 'efficiency' describes the ability to perform an action and bring about the desired result. Also, in physics 'efficiency' means the amount of energy or work put in to produce a result. The less efficient a process the more work/energy is needed to attain the same end.

Translated into general practice 'efficiency' describes how well a practice fulfils its aims (whatever they are) and how much energy and time is needed to do so. If two practices share the same aim of giving all children registered with them their preschool booster the efficient practice will have a higher uptake and have a system of recall which absorbs less staff time than a less efficient one. If two practices believe that patient satisfaction is important then the more efficient will ensure that the way they run their systems will enhance rather than diminish patient satisfaction. We do not believe there is a conflict between efficiency and caritas. If efficiency and caritas appear to conflict we suggest 'caritas' is not a real objective within the practice.

Factors Affecting Efficiency

One way of representing what happens in general practice is shown in Figure 26.1. In this figure it is suggested that the ability to run a practice efficiently depends on premises which should be well designed and suited for the purpose, on staff and partners who should know what their jobs are, perform them well and be satisfied with their working conditions, and on systems which are each designed for a specific purpose. In order to know what is happening it is necessary to have feedback with or without analysis. The one major factor missing in this figure is the ability to change (see Figure 26.2) which must be present before any improvements can take place.

Figure 26.1: Schematic Representation of General Practice

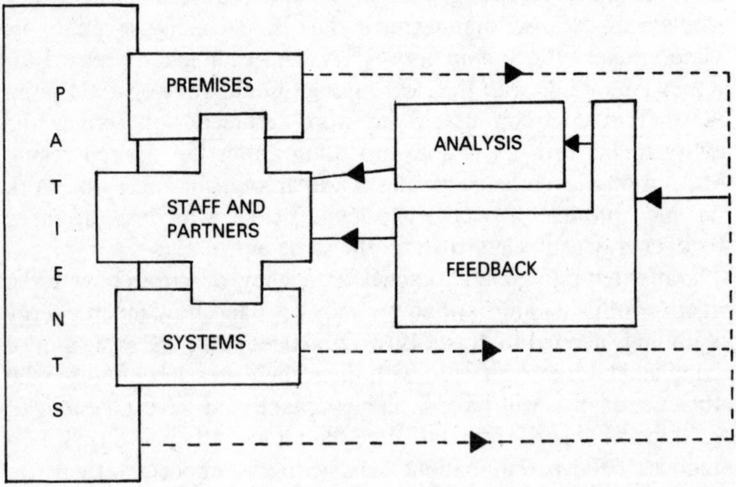

Figure 26.2: Change and Feedback

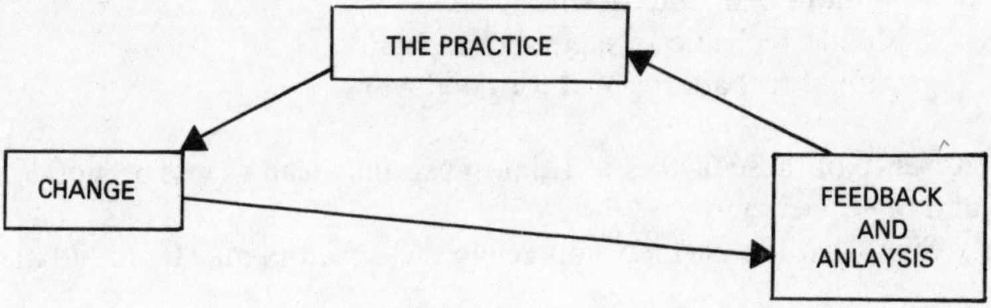

Blocks in the system which impair efficiency may occur at any stage; staff may not understand their roles, or be employed in a job which is too easy or difficult for them. They may be underpaid. Partners themselves may not understand the roles of employed or attached staff. Systems may not work, but in the absence of feedback may get snarled up, with patients suffering in silence. The mechanism of feedback and analysis may exist — but how often is the analysis left unused causing mounting frustration among those who spend time and energy maintaining it. The practice as a whole may be so rigid or unco-ordinated that even when the need for change becomes obvious nothing happens. With efficient management such blocks should not occur. They should be prevented. If they do arise they should be recognised.

Conditions Needed for a Healthy Organisation

In the previous section an overall view was given of the main factors involved in running a practice efficiently. In this section the individual components will be looked at in greater detail.

1. Staff

In order to maintain good morale and motivation it is necessary that staff

a . capabilities should match the job;
b. personality should match the practice;
c. should be aware of their own and others' roles;

d. should be fairly paid and feel secure;
e. should feel able to report back on the working of the practice without being put down;
f. should feel able to suggest change;
g. should feel appreciated for good work.

Absence of these factors will almost certainly lead to loss of morale and of efficiency.

Signs that the partners appreciate these factors may be found in

1. definition of a careful appointment process;
2. appropriate referrals by receptionists and others to, for example, the practice nurse or health visitor;
3. an explicit wage structure with a mechanism for annual review;
4. availability of staff contracts;
5. existence of clear rules which are understood, and of written procedures;
6. defined responsibilities and lines of responsibility;
7. evidence of changes in systems suggested by staff;
8. low staff turnover, cheerful atmosphere, good morale (evinced by attitude and personal touches in staff working areas);
9. staff-generated social activities.

2. Partners

We suggest that in order to maintain harmonious working relationships, with each partner carrying his/her fair share of work and responsibility, partners should:

a. receive what each considers a fair division of profit for work done;
b. agree arrangements for holidays and off-duty;
c. agree on the aims to be pursued and systems to be used within the practice;
d. participate in shared decisions on all partnership matters.

Among the signs that partners acknowledge that these factors are important would be:

1. the existence of a partnership agreement;

2. a low turnover of partners, especially junior partners or assistants;
3. statements of agreed practice policy;
4. the recording of shared decisions.

3. Premises

In order to promote efficiency we suggest that premises should:

a. be of adequate size;
b. suit the purposes of the practice;
c. be funded (and improved) by the most advantageous method.

Signs that the partners are aware that the efficiency of the practice is affected by the premises from which they practice are:

1. provision of adequate space, furnishings and equipment in good repair for all the functions undertaken in the practice;
2. evidence of appreciation of the need for sound proofing and privacy for both patients and staff;
3. use of appropriate improvement grants and rent reimbursements.

4. Systems

The characteristics of successful systems are considered in detail in Chapter 22. Evidence that partners appreciate the importance of these characteristics may be found if:

1. systems have stated purposes;
2. systems have written procedures;
3. staff can describe what they do and why;
4. staff can demonstrate that a monitoring system exists to show whether the system is succeeding in its purpose or not.

Feedback, Decisions and Change

Even when all the conditions we have described for staff, partners, premises and systems are met the organisation of the practice may stagnate, the practice may not be able to adapt to changing circumstances. This will happen:

1. If the Practice is Unaware of its Position

We have stressed the need for feedback on individual systems. If, however, the partners remain ignorant of the overall state of their practice they have no basis on which to plan changes. They cannot know where to go because they do not know where they are. One way of avoiding this is for the partners to hold an annual review of all facets of the practice, its staff and its organisation.

2. If There is No Mechanism for Decision-making and for Ensuring that Decisions are Followed by Action

One of the commonest failures in management in general practice is to talk round a subject, to agree that something should be done — and to do nothing about it. The failure may arise for a number of reasons. A firm decision may not be made. No agreement may have been reached as to how the decision is to be put into practice. The responsibility for ensuring that action is taken may not be assigned to anyone. The only way to avoid this problem is for decisions to be written down, responsibility assigned, and an automatic check that action has been taken after a specified time interval instituted.

3. If the Partners and Practice are Incapable of Change

Everyone involved with the practice, patients, staff and practice, will be affected by changes over time. Individuals react differently to change. Some will welcome and accept, some will be indifferent, others will resist either actively or passively. Reactions vary according to the individual, the changes proposed, and the way that the changes are introduced. There is a considerable body of business management literature concerned with the management of change. Common sense dictates that if the people involved are consulted early, understand the reasoning behind the proposed change and share in the planning, resistance will be diminished and discussion will tend to be constructive rather than destructive.

Envoie

In this chapter we have spelt out the fact that management in general practice involves premises, systems and, most importantly, people. We have discussed management principles and have suggested that practitioners examine their own practices against this background.

Until recently the importance of management, which we see as complementary rather than accessary to clinical care, has been underestimated in general practice. We believe that a change of attitude is discernible in the profession. We hope the material we have presented will accelerate that change. Good management has to be worked at, it doesn't just happen.

APPENDIX I: CHOOSING A PRACTICE

> Variety's the very spice of life,
> That gives it all its flavour.
>
> William Cowper

Choosing a practice has been likened to choosing a marriage partner and indeed there are a number of similarities. If the choice is successful then the relationship can be long, happy and rewarding, both emotionally and financially. If the choice is incompatible then the results can be disastrous with acrimony, unhappiness, and considerable financial loss on all sides.

Therefore, a great deal of thought and care must go into choosing a practice and partners who suit your particular temperament and family needs. Most young doctors have a fantasy of the ideal practice. It would be in a pleasant area, near the sea and good recreational facilities but with a first-class district general hospital at hand and in premises bulging with modern gadgetry and ancillary staff! Indeed a survey of vocational trainees undertaken a few years ago showed that a large percentage hoped for a medium-sized market-town practice with purpose-built premises in a rural part of the country. Unfortunately, there are not enough ideal practices around to suit everybody and this fantasy must be tempered by reality.

There is a great deal to be said for young doctors gaining experience of different types of practice before committing themselves. This experience can be obtained either in the trainee year in general practice (when the whole time does not have to be spent in one practice), or by doing a variety of locums in different areas and types of practice. If possible, it is worth trying to spend some time in groups, and also in single-handed practice; there are considerable differences between the two which are difficult to appreciate unless both have been experienced.

The single-handed practice is becoming less common. The present trend, encouraged by government, is towards group practice. However, there will always be a place for the individual practitioner in parts of the country where the population is not dense enough to support more than one doctor. There are also those doctors who, by temperament, are better suited to single-handed practice.

A group practice provides more variety of experience amongst the doctors and decreases the risk of professional isolation. Duty rotas in groups means that a doctor is less frequently on call, but usually when on duty he is busier because of the larger number of patients for which he is responsible.

In a very large practice the incoming doctor may find it difficult to 'make his mark'. He may find himself having to bow to majority verdicts in practice decisions which may frustrate him if there are certain aspects of the practice which he would like to change.

In choosing a practice a difficulty which may seem surprising is the wide range of possibilities that the aspiring general practitioner has to choose from. But if during training the doctor has had experience of a variety of types of practice — urban, rural, single and groups — he should have some idea of the type and location of practice in which he is interested. A check list of the main factors which vary between one practice and another is given in Section 2. Reference to this list may help to define priorities.

When the search for a practice begins, the best source of information is still the 'bush telegraph'. Chance enquiries started in this way can often bear fruit. This is particularly true for trainees during their three-year vocational courses, because they have ample opportunity to meet local general practitioners during their stay in an area and their general practitioner trainer may also know of local vacancies. Course organisers, too, receive enquiries from local general practitioners seeking new partners.

Other services include advertising in the *British Medical Journal (BMJ)*, and in the *Journal of the Royal College of General Practitioners (JRCGP)* and in medical newspapers. The *BMJ* also runs a special service (The Medical Practices Bureau) for members to find practices and it is worth writing to Tavistock Square for the latest details of practices in specific localities. Not all the practice vacancies on their records are advertised in the *BMJ*. The local BMA offices are also always very helpful, and willing to give advice about vacancies.

One of the fascinations of visiting practices is that they are all so different. It is impossible to do anything more than generalise about the points to consider. However, the prospective partner might like to consider some of the following items:

1. The Partners

What are their ages and interests? How do they relate to each other and to you? Do they seem flexible in their ideas and not unwilling to modify their attitudes and habits if a good case can be made for doing so? Have there been any recent partnership changes and, if so, why? Indeed, why has the practice vacancy arisen at all? Are the partners members of the Royal College of General Practitioners and, if not, what are their attitudes to the College? Are any of the partners trainers in a vocational training scheme? If not, are they at all interested in teaching? If there is a trainee in the practice, it would be certainly worthwhile trying to get him on his own to talk about the practice. Not many doctors are interested in research or in writing learned papers but if a partner is involved in research or has written papers then it again suggests that the practice may accommodate flexible interests. Do they have other outside interests, for example, medico-political, college activities, or Rotary?

In the past, the term 'senior partner' often meant not only the oldest member of the practice but also the doctor who had the right of veto in practice activities. He might have less out-of-hours work and take the greatest share of the profits. This is less so now, and the term 'senior partner' usually only refers to the doctor who has been in the practice the longest. It is important to see that a retirement clause is written into the partnership agreement so that the situation does not arise whereby an elderly doctor, out of touch with reality, refuses to retire. This clause should be written in such a way that, if the retiring partner wishes to go on working, he can then be re-employed, perhaps on a salary basis with less work and responsibility.

2. The Premises

Are they in a health centre or privately owned, purpose-built or adapted? If privately owned, what financial commitment will the incoming partner have to meet? If the premises seem inadequate, are there possibilities of addition, alterations or removal to more suitable ones in the future? Does each doctor have his own room and, if not, does the timetable of the practice allow each doctor to run his surgery within a reasonable period of time without too much pressure to vacate the room for the next doctor? Does the practice have a nurse and if so has she an adequate treatment-room? What is the practice policy about items of equipment, such as the ECG or basic furniture? Does the practice have a library? If so, are the books about general practice? Look at the records as they can reveal much about the practice's standard of medical care.

3. The Workload

Is the work shared evenly between the partners, including the rota duties? If partners have special commitments, such as clinical assistantships, who covers the practice while they are away? If one partner consults at a rate of, say, 12 per hour and another partner consults at a slower rate, will this cause argument and misunderstanding? What holiday arrangements are made? It is usual now for partners to have about six weeks holiday a year and this may or may not include study leave. Some practices now also include arrangements in their agreements for sabbatical leave, for example, six months every eight years. This is a subject worth discussing. When a partner is on holiday, are there adequate arrangements for covering his work?

4. Parity

The average length of time until parity of income is achieved is usually about three years with an agreed percentage sliding scale until this time. For example, in a three-man practice an incoming partner might start at 25 per cent for the first year, 28 per cent for the second year and 30 per cent for the third year with an equal one third share after this. Some doctors resent the concept of working towards parity, but one must remember that the other partners have built up the practice and the incoming doctor reaps the benefit. Attitudes are perhaps easier to understand if one remembers that twenty years ago it was not uncommon for young partners to wait ten years or more for parity! As a general rule it tends to be the case that popular practices in a pleasant area can ask an incoming partner to work more time to parity than would be expected in an overstretched city centre practice. It is normal for a new entrant to a practice to work for a specified period of time, anything from three months to a year, with an easy break clause in the contract. This is to the advantage of both sides. It means that if it is mutually agreed that the appointment was a mistake, then separation is easier. This initial period may be in the form of a salaried assistantship or partnership.

5. Partnership Agreements

All partnerships should have an agreement, if only to be agreed and put away. The various aspects of this agreement have been discussed in Chapter 12. Beware of the partnership which says, 'Oh, we don't need an agreement!'

6. Flexibility

Flexibility and a willingness to consider new ideas are qualities in a partnership and practice which will be of interest to all aspiring new partners. It is particularly important for married women practitioners whose family commitments may dictate their pattern of work, sometimes at short notice.

Evidence that the practice is capable of altering its organisation to meet changing circumstances may be sought by asking what changes have been instituted in the last few years and by enquiring about plans for the future.

7. Income

Money has been dealt with in detail in Chapters 16 to 20. It has been deliberately left low in the order of priorities when considering a practice. If income is the only matter of interest then probably the young doctor will be seeking a post overseas and not reading this book! Naturally money is important, but too much emphasis can be laid upon it. The average income of a well-trained new entrant to practice will probably be in the region of £12,000-£16,000 in the first year (1984 figures). It is essential to have a look at the practice accounts and get some idea of the potential income of the practice and what earnings will be at parity rather than be over-concerned with the starting figure. Enquire about the distribution of non-NHS earnings, such as private examinations, cremation fees, factory appointments, clinical assistantships, and so on. The fairest way is for all the practice income to be pooled and divided equally amongst the partners according to their shares. Any other method may lead to problems and even to the break-up of the partnership unless all partners feel happy with the arrangements. Nevertheless, it is quite common for partners to keep their own seniority award, and vocational training allowance. However, if this happens, it is important to see that no ill-will occurs as a result. Further advice about information which can be gleaned from the practice accounts is given in Chapter 19.

8. Housing

This will vary according to need but it is as well to have some idea of how much a suitable house in the area would cost. It is worth enquiring whether it would be possible to rent accommodation for some months while settling into the practice and getting to know the area. Some practices like the junior partner to live on the premises and although this habit is now dying out, it is as well to be aware of it.

9. Schools

Doctors with present or future young families forget that children need schools surprisingly quickly. Unless children are to be sent to boarding schools it is important to look at the local primary and secondary schools to find out what they have to offer.

The Interview

All these points will need to be discussed when the doctor goes to the practice for an interview. However, before this stage he will need to write to the practice concerned either applying for the post or asking for further details. In doing this it is important to create a good impression. Handwriting should be legible and a typed curriculum vitae is preferable. The curriculum vitae should be fairly brief with a mention of secondary education and medical school. Give more detail about postgraduate experience indicating special qualifications where appropriate (e.g. FP certificate). State if married, wife's occupation (if any) and family (if any). Finally add hobbies and special interests (non-medical) since these help to build a more complete picture of you as an individual.

References will be required and these should be carefully selected. If a general practitioner knows you well, for example a trainer or family doctor, then use him. General practitioners tend not to be over impressed with vague references from grandiose consultants in teaching hospitals. Remember to contact your referees to ask their permission to use their names. It is also useful to referees if you give them a quick outline of the practice to which you are applying.

Having been short-listed and asked for interview, the procedure may now vary a little. Many doctors like to entertain prospective partners and their wives for the day as this is often the best way to assess each other in surroundings which are fairly informal. It is unwise for a married doctor not to have taken his spouse to the practice before the final decision is made and they should ask if they can do this if not invited to do so. Indeed a practice where the wife was not invited would be suspect. Try to meet all the partners on this visit and remember that you are assessing them and their practice as much as they are assessing you.

Most practices expect to pay interview expenses. If they are not offered enquire about them as it will give a guide to practice attitudes on finance.

After the first visit, if both sides are interested in pursuing matters further, at least one more visit will be needed before a decision is taken. Do not rush into making a hasty decision because the area seems attractive or the premises are good. The main thing that really matters is the compatability of the partners and yourself. If this is wrong then it will never work out. If it is right then with goodwill on all sides almost any other problem can be resolved. When in doubt about particular aspects, keep making enquiries and do not try to ignore them in the hope that they will go away. They never do.

Section 2: Practice Check List

The following check list is suggested as an *aide-mémoire* of questions to be asked when visiting a practice. If several practices are visited it may aid comparison if each question is scored 0-5, the highest total score showing the practice which is nearest your own ideal.

1. Partners

(a) Age. Sex. Seniority.
(b) Attitudes to each other.
(c) Attitudes to wives (including yours).
(d) Attitudes to the RCGP.
(e) Special interests.
(f) Research and/or publications.
(g) Flexibility of approach.
(h) Reason for partnership vacancy.

2. Premises

(a) Health centre.
(b) Privately owned — what is incoming partner's financial commitment?
(c) Adequate space.
(d) Own consulting-room.
(e) Employed staff — receptionists, etc.
(f) Employed practice nurse.
(g) Attached staff (D/N, H/V, Social worker).
(h) Equipment, e.g. ECG.
(i) Furnishing and general impression.
(j) Any special features.
(k) Record system — quality of records.
(l) Staff room.
(m) Age-sex register.

3. Partnership Agreement

(a) Is there one?
(b) Time to parity.
(c) Restrictive clauses.

4. Money

(a) Partnership accounts.

(b) Outside income, e.g. clinical assistantships.
(c) Is all income shared equally?
(d) Situation re seniority allowance, VT allowance, etc.
(e) Are employed staff paid realistic salaries?
(f) Is money being spent on improving the quality of care (e.g. pleasant premises, equipment, etc.)?

5. *Workload*

(a) Is work shared evenly?
(b) Is off-duty rota satisfactory?
(c) Is there an appointment system?
(d) Does the practice seem under pressure?
(e) Is there scope for expansion, e.g. clinical assistantship sessions, teaching, etc?
(f) Do the wives have to cover the telephone except when on call?

6. *Holidays*

(a) Amount per year.
(b) Study leave allowance.
(c) Restrictive clauses, e.g. only one partner away at a time.
(d) Sabbatical arrangements.

7. *Housing*

8. *Schools*

It must be emphasised that this list does not necessarily mean that items included are good or, if excluded, bad. It is purely an *aide-mémoire* and a help towards personal selection.

APPENDIX II: USEFUL ADDRESSES

The Practice

1. Association of Medical Secretaries,
   Tavistock House South, Tavistock Square,
   London WC1H 9LN

   Tel. No. 01-387-6005

2. Association of Health Centres and Practice Administrators.
   121 Woodgrange Road, Forest Hill,
   Forest Gate, London E7 0EP

   Tel. No. 01-555-5331

3. Central Information Service,
   Royal College of General Practitioners,
   14 Princes Gate,
   London SW7 1PU

   Tel. No. 01-584-3232

   This service has recently been renamed The RCGP Information Service.

4. General Medical Council,
   44 Hallam Street, London W1N 6AE

   Tel. No. 01-580-7642

5. General Practice Finance Corporation,
   Tavistock House North, Tavistock Square,
   London WC1 9JL

   Tel. No. 01-387-5274

6. Medical Practices Committee, England and Wales,
   Tavistock House South, Tavistock Square,
   London WC1

   Tel. No. 01-388-6471

   Scotland: St. Andrew's House, Edinburgh EH1 3DI

   Tel. No. 031-556-8501

Associations and Colleges

7. Association of Police Surgeons of Great Britain,
Creaton House, Creaton,
Northampton NN6 8ND

Tel. No. 060-124-744

8. British Medical Association,
General Medical Services Committee,
including the Trainee's Sub-committee,
Personal Services Bureau,
Medical Practices Advisory Bureau,
BMA House, Tavistock Square,
London WC1H 9JP

Tel. No. 01-387-4499

9. Medico-Legal Society,
33 Henrietta Street,
Strand, London WC2E 8NH

Tel. No. 01-836 0011

10. Medical Officers of Schools Association,
The Secretary,
Eton Court House, Eton,
Windsor, Berkshire SL4 6AQ

Tel. No. 075-35-64678

11. Medical Practitioners Union/ASTMS,
79 Camden Road, London NW1 9ES

Tel. No. 01-267-4422

12. Medical Women's Federation,
Tavistock House North, Tavistock Square,
London WC1H 9HX

Tel. No. 01-387-7765

13. Royal College of General Practitioners,
14 Princes Gate,
London SW7 1PU

Tel. No. 01-584-3232

14. Society of Occupational Medicine,
    c/o Royal College of Physicians,
    11 St. Andrew's Place, London NW1 4LE

    Tel. No. 01-486-2641

GP Research and Postgraduate Activities

15. British Postgraduate Medical Federation,
    (University of London),
    14 Millman Mews, Millman Street,
    London WC1 3EJ

    Tel. No. 01-831-6222

16. Council for Postgraduate Medical Education,
    England and Wales,
    7 Marylebone Road, London NW1 5HA

    Tel. No. 01-323-1289

    N. Ireland: 5 Annadale Avenue, Belfast BT7 3JH

    Tel. No. 0232-640731

    Scotland: 8 Queen Square, Edinburgh EH2 1JE

    Tel. No. 031-255-4365

17. Medical Research Council,
    20 Park Crescent, London W1N 4AL

    Tel. No. 01-636-4365

Defence Bodies

18. The Medical Defence Union Ltd.,
    3 Devonshire Place, London W1N 2EA

    Tel. No. 01-486 6181

19. The Medical Protection Society Ltd.,
    50 Hallam Street, London W1N 6DE

    Tel. No. 01-637-0541

20. The Medical and Dental Defence Union of Scotland Ltd.,
113 St. Vincent Street,
Glasgow

Tel. No. 041-221-8381

Government Departments

21. Department of Health and Social Security,
Alexander Fleming House,
Elephant & Castle, London SE1 6BY

Tel. No. 01-407-5522

22. Northern Ireland: Department of Health and Social Services,
Dundonald House, Upper Newtownards Road, Belfast BT4 3SF

Tel. No. 0232-650111

23. Scottish Home and Health Department,
St. Andrew's House, Edinburgh EH1 3DI

Tel. No. 031-556-8501

24. Welsh Office: Health and Social Work Department,
New Crown Building, Cathays Park, Cardiff CF1 3NQ

Tel. No. 0222-825111

25. HM Stationery Office,
Administration,
Britannia House, 7 Trinity Street,
London SE1

Tel. No. 01-928-8933

INDEX